THE WAY TO PEACE

*Love to Judy,
One of the most
"peace-full" people
I know.*

*Sanderson Beck, the
author, is a good
friend of our son's
family, and also of
me and Joe. He was
the speaker at a Beyond
War workshop in Great Falls.
He lives in Ojai, California
now.*

Sanderson Beck was born March 5, 1947 in Los Angeles. He received a B.A. in Dramatic Art from the University of California at Berkeley, an M.A. in Religious Studies from U.C. Santa Barbara, Ph.D. candidacy in the Philosophy of Education from U.C.L.A., and a Ph.D. in Philosophy from the World University. He was ordained a Minister of Light and initiated by John-Roger in 1972. Sanderson now lives in Ojai, California where he has taught at the World University since 1976. He is also on the faculty of International College, which offers independent studies tutorials. In 1982 he formulated World Peace Movement Principles, Purposes, and Methods. The plan for the first nine volumes of his collected works is as follows:

1. *Religious Studies*
2. *Papers on Education*
3. *Collected Screenplays*
4. *Confucius and Socrates*
5. *The Good Message of Jesus the Christ*
6. *The Soul*
7. *The Way to Peace*
8. *Peace Writings*
9. *Principles of Education*

THE WAY TO PEACE

The Great Peacemakers
Philosophers of Peace
and Efforts toward World Peace

by Sanderson Beck

Coleman Publishing
99 Milbar Boulevard
Farmingdale, New York 11735

Coleman Publishing
99 Milbar Blvd.
Farmingdale, N.Y. 11735

First printing February, 1986
Manufactured in the United States of America
Cover design by Coleman Publishing

ISBN 0-87418-037-6

Dedicated
to all those
who are working for peace and justice
in peaceful, loving ways

CONTENTS

Introduction

Over a century ago, Victor Hugo wrote that one can resist the invasion of armies but not the power of ideas whose time has come. What the world needs now more than ever is a way to establish lasting peace. The military build-up of the last few years has awakened public cries of concern and protest. The danger of a nuclear war has become the most important issue of the eighties, for it concerns the very survival of our civilization. Much has been written about the problems of nuclear weapons, military intervention, economic burdens, and the cold war. Discussions of solutions to these problems have tended to focus on short-term remedies such as a bilateral nuclear weapons freeze. Ultimately we must discover and apply deeper and more enduring solutions as well. Understanding permanent solutions to our dilemma gives an invaluable perspective and encouragement toward facing this horrendous situation.

The philosophy of peacemaking has been evolving through the centuries and can be found in all the great cultures of the world. The way of peace has been practiced and taught by ancient sages and founders of religions, such as Lao Tzu, Confucius, Mahavira, the Buddha, Pythagoras, Socrates, Jesus, and Bahá'u'lláh. Their messages have been carried by peacemakers like Mencius, St. Francis of Assisi, Chaucer, Erasmus, George Fox, and many others. Principles of justice through international law have been taught by Dante, Crucé, Grotius, Penn, Rousseau, Bentham, Kant, and Emerson. Methods of nonviolent civil disobedience have been passed directly from Thoreau to Tolstoy to Gandhi to King. In our war-torn twentieth century, evolving experiments with limited world government are seen in the League of Nations and the United Nations and in recent proposals for more effective world law. Great philosophers and pacifists such as Einstein, Schweitzer, Russell, and Muste have protested nuclear weapons. The tragedy of the Vietnam War stimulated the first peace movement that was able to stop a major war. The modern feminist movement has increased people's awareness of the role of women in bringing balance and peace to

society. In the eighties a movement opposed to nuclear technology has grown and is striving for a nuclear-free world. *The Way to Peace* is the story of their efforts to make peace and their insights into the psychological, social, political, and economic factors of war and peace, the root causes of war, and how to transform society into a peaceful world.

He shall judge between the nations,
and shall decide for many peoples;
and they shall beat their swords into plowshares,
and their spears into pruning hooks;
nation shall not lift up sword against nation,
neither shall they learn war any more.

Isaiah 2:4

1
Chinese Sages: Lao Tzu, Confucius, Mo Tzu, and Mencius

"Whoever loves the world as his self
may be entrusted to care for the world."

Lao Tzu

"If men were to regard the states of others
as they regard their own,
then who would raise up his state
to attack the state of another?"

Mo Tzu

Lao Tzu lived in China in the sixth century B.C. Historical records indicate that he was the Keeper of the Archives in the imperial capital at Loyang. Legend tells us that when he was old and tired of the corruption of the world he rode an ox-drawn chariot to the mountain pass of the western frontier. The Keeper of the Pass, having observed omens in the weather and expecting a sage, begged the old man to write a book before withdrawing from civilization. So Lao Tzu composed the *Tao Teh Ching,* consisting of about 5,250 Chinese characters (words). This concise book is probably one of the greatest writings in the world and became the scriptural foundation of the Taoist religion. *Tao* means the way and implies an absolute reality roughly comparable to the Western idea of God; yet it is described not anthropomorphically but as a dynamic and natural process. *Teh* means virtue in the sense of spiritual power. *Ching* is the word for book or classic.

In the *Tao Teh Ching* Lao Tzu describes a simple, natural, and peaceful way of life. Serenity may be found by returning to the eternal source, by emptying oneself of all desires, and by flowing like water. The universe has two complementary principles — the male *(yang)* and the female *(yin).* Harmony results from the natural balance of the active and receptive qualities. Those who are too aggressive meddle in their affairs and cause unnecessary problems, while those who are too passive lose their center and fail to maintain a natural order. Since the human tendency is to

1

be too active and interfering, Lao Tzu emphasizes the inward process of action through non-action *(wu-wei).* By being receptive to this transcendental way, one knows intuitively how much to do and when to stop. The primary responsibility of each person is to understand and master oneself.

Whoever knows others is wise.
Whoever knows himself is enlightened.
Whoever conquers others has physical strength.
Whoever conquers himself is strong.
Whoever is content is wealthy.
Whoever is determined has strong will.
Whoever does not lose his center endures.
Whoever dies but maintains his spiritual power has eternal life.

The way of spiritual power never interferes or inflicts, yet through it everything is accomplished; for it is the essence of what is. All we need to do is to follow the way things are, and the world will be reformed of its own accord. The conflict of personal desires is what obscures the way, but when we free ourselves of desire then we find peace. The way that works best for all is a transcendental but dynamic, living reality which we can easily follow by understanding our own nature.

In political life Lao Tzu also recommended following this transcendental way. The idea that "the violent die a violent death" he made the foundation of his teaching. Violence opposes the way of living, and whatever opposes life will soon perish. The use of force tends to rebound, and when armies march the country is laid to waste. Whenever a large army is raised, scarcity and want follow. The more weapons the state has, the more trouble there will be. It is better to withdraw than to attack. One should not under-estimate one's enemy, and it is possible to confront them and win them over without fighting them. When there is a battle, those who are kind truly win. A good leader is not violent; a good fighter does not get angry; a good winner is not vengeful; a good employer is humble. This is the heavenly way of dealing with people. Loving mercy brings courage and victory; economy brings abundance and generosity; and humility brings natural leadership. Heaven gives loving mercy to those it would not see destroyed. Whoever knows how to preserve life

2

with these qualities will not be harmed by wild animals nor wounded in battle, because there is no death in him. The one who is brave in fighting will be killed, but the one who is brave in not fighting will live. People are not afraid of death, so why threaten them with it? How can we judge who is evil and to be killed? There is a master executioner who regulates death, and if someone attempts to undertake His work he rarely escapes without injuring himself. Living things are tender and flexible, but dead things are stiff and rigid; thus an inflexible government will be defeated. A large country is like the lower part of a river where the waters converge; it can win over small countries by placing itself below them, and a small country can win over a large country by serving it.

The teachings of Confucius (551-479 B.C.) harmonize well with those of Lao Tzu. While the approach of Lao Tzu was mystical, Confucius emphasized ethics and social philosophy. Confucius was the first well-known professional teacher in ancient China, and he served occasionally as a political advisor to princes. Through the influence of Confucius' teachings it became possible for men to rise in social position by educating themselves and developing their abilities. Confucius was born into the lower aristocratic class of the impoverished knights. By the age of fifteen he had decided to concentrate on learning and the improvement of his character. By the age of fifty he felt that he knew what the Will of Heaven was for him. He advised the local ruler on good government. When asked if it would help those following the Way to kill those who were not following the Way, Confucius responded, "You are there to rule, not to kill. If you desire what is good, the people will at once be good." When he found that his principles were not really being put into practice he traveled to other states looking for a ruler who would listen to his advice. When the Duke of Wei asked his advice on military strategy, Confucius replied that he had not studied warfare; he left Wei the next day. While he was journeying through Sung, Huan T'ui, the Minister of War in that state, attempted to assassinate him. Confucius' confidence was not shaken, for he said, "Heaven produced the virtue that is in me. What do I have to fear from such a one as Huan T'ui?" Apparently Confucius did not hold this incident against Huan T'ui's brother Ssu-ma Niu, because he accepted Ssu-ma Niu as one of his regular students. Although eager to give political advice, Confucius twice renounced invitations by rulers, because they were involved in civil wars. Returning to Wei to advise the ruling minister there, Confucius was asked by the minister how he might go about attacking a noble who had offended the minister's daughter. Confucius told him not to attack, but when the minister went ahead with it, Confucius prepared his chariot to leave. When the minister apologized, Confucius was ready to stay, but then messengers arrived inviting him to return to his home state of Lu.

Confucius taught that a person ought to make his own conduct correct before he attempts to correct or rule over others. The ruler is analogous to the parent whose first obligation is to love the children; therefore the ruler must love the people. The people are to be loyal to the ruler, but for Confucius this loyalty means admonishing the leaders when they do wrong. Everyone is responsible for one's own actions. Confucius said, "The commander of three armies may be taken away, but the will of even a common man may not be taken away from him." The essence of Confucius' teachings is humanity *(jen)*. Goodness is the action of loving people, and wisdom is found in understanding people. Perhaps the teachings of Confucius regarding inner peace and peace in society can best be summarized by the brief Confucian classic attributed to him entitled *Higher Education*.

> The Way of higher education is cultivated and practiced by
>   manifesting the enlightening character of spiritual power,
>   loving the people as they grow,
>   and living in the highest good.
> By knowing and living in the highest good, purpose is directed.
> When purpose is directed, one becomes calm.
> When one is calm, then peace can be found.
> In peace, one may contemplate.
> Through contemplation, the goal is attained.
> Living things have their roots and branches;
> Human events have their beginnings and endings.

4

To understand what is first and last will lead one near the Way.
The ancients who wished to manifest
   the enlightening character of spiritual power to the world
   would first bring order to their government.
Wishing to bring order to their government,
   they would first regulate their communities.
Wishing to regulate their communities,
   they would first cultivate their personal lives.
Wishing to cultivate their personal lives,
   they would first set their hearts right.
Wishing to set their hearts right,
   they would first make their wills sincere.
Wishing to make their wills sincere,
   they would first extend their knowledge to the utmost.
Extension of knowledge comes from the investigation of things.
When things are investigated, knowledge is extended.
When knowledge is extended, the will becomes sincere.
When the will is sincere, the heart can be set right.
When the heart is right, the personal life can be cultivated.
When the personal life is cultivated,
   the community can be regulated.
When the community is regulated,
   the government can be made orderly.
And when the government is orderly,
   there will be peace in the world.
From the Son of Heaven down to the common people,
   all must consider cultivation of the personal life as the root.
There cannot be a disordered root growing into ordered branches.
If what is near is neglected,
   how can one take care of what is far away?
This is the root and foundation of knowledge.

Mo Tzu lived in the fifth century B.C. after the death of
Confucius. He studied under the scholars of the growing
Confucian school, but he became an independent religious
teacher with several hundred devoted disciples who were willing
to follow him anywhere. Living ascetically and preaching
universal love he criticized the Confucian philosophy for its

5

excessive use of rituals, elaborate funerals and music, and what he believed to be its fatalism. Moism challenged Confucianism for prominence in China for two hundred years until it was somehow demolished during the violent Ch'in empire. For most of its history since then China was influenced by Confucianism, Taoism, and Buddhism. Perhaps Mo Tzu's philosophy of universal love without distinction was too idealistic for a culture that was so loyal to family ties.

Mo Tzu and his disciples traveled from place to place preaching and attempting to prevent wars. When Mo Tzu heard that Kung Shu Pan had constructed ladders so that he could attack the small state of Sung, he walked ten days and ten nights, tearing off pieces of his garment to wrap his feet, in order to talk with Kung Shu Pan. Mo Tzu began by asking Kung Shu Pan to kill someone in the north who had humiliated him. Kung Shu Pan declared that murder was against his principles. Whereupon Mo Tzu bowed in apology and explained that for a ruler of a large state to attack a small and innocent state was also against the principle of killing. When Kung Shu Pan argued that he had already promised his king he would attack, Mo Tzu asked to be presented to the king. He asked the king why one who has so much would try to steal from one who has little. The king mentioned the ladders, but Mo Tzu laid out a model city and showed how he with only a small stick could defend the city against Kung Shu Pan's machines. Aware that the king was thinking he could murder him, Mo Tzu declared that three hundred of his disciples were waiting on the city wall of Sung with implements of defense. Even though Mo Tzu might be killed, the city could not be taken. Thereupon the king decided not to attack.

One man once challenged Mo Tzu that his idea of universal love did not benefit the world and this man's not loving the world did no harm. Mo Tzu posed a parable: If there was a terrible fire, and one man fetched water to extinguish it and another fuel to reinforce it, even though neither had yet accomplished anything, which one was more valuable? Thus the intention to love universally was better than the opposite.

Mo Tzu exhorted people to be virtuous for the good that it would do for all. He said, "Let him who has strength be alert to help others; let him who has wealth endeavor to share it with others; let him who possesses the Way teach others persuasively. With this, the hungry will be fed, the cold will be clothed, the disturbed will have peace . . . This is procuring abundant life." However, too often the rulers honored relatives, the rich, and the goodlooking rather than those with merit. Mo Tzu suggested that people identify with Heaven which is universally beneficial. The one who obeys the will of Heaven practices righteousness, but the one who uses force is disobeying the will of Heaven. When righteousness is followed, the strong will not oppress the weak, the eminent will not lord it over the humble, and the cunning will not deceive the stupid. Mo Tzu transcended political authority when he said that people must go beyond identifying with the Son of Heaven (Emperor) and identify with Heaven itself.

For Mo Tzu the universal-minded person loves his friend the same as himself, and his friend's father the same as his own. Thus he will feed him when he is hungry, clothe him when he is cold, take care of him when he is sick, and bury him when he dies. Would it be wiser to entrust one's parents to such a universal-minded person or to one who is partial? Likewise rulers ought to care for their subjects in the same way, and government ought to treat another state the same as its own state. Such a government would never attack another state. By not threatening other states they would be left in peace, and by reducing military expenditures prosperity would result. Mo Tzu believed that warfare as mass murder was that much more of a crime than a single murder, and yet often people praise war and call it righteous. Murdering men is hardly the way to benefit them, and the expenditures of warfare cripple the nation's livelihood and exhaust the resources of the people. During war the affairs of government are neglected, the farms lie fallow, and many of the best men are lost. Mo Tzu concludes, "Such is the injury which warfare inflicts upon men, the harm it brings to the world. And yet the rulers and officials delight in carrying out such expeditions. In effect they are taking delight in the injury and extermination of the people of the world. Are they not perverse?"

Mencius (371-289 B.C.) studied under Confucius' grandson's pupil, and his writings became one of the Confucian classics. Like Confucius he was a professional teacher and a political advisor who traveled from state to state. Mencius believed that human nature is innately good and that we need only discover the heart. He criticized Mo Tzu's doctrine of universal love without distinctions, advocating humanity with a righteousness that discerns the proper distinctions in human relationships. He recommended humane government and felt that righteousness is far more important than utility and profit. Mencius believed that virtue is inherent in everyone's nature and that therefore everyone is equal to everyone else; also the people are most important in the state, and they have the right to change their government.

A humane government places men of virtue and ability in positions of responsibility and works to benefit the people; such a country will be at peace and free of troubles. Mencius pointed out that when men are subdued by force their hearts are not won over and they only submit because they are not able to resist, but when they are won over by virtue their hearts are pleased and their cooperation is sincere. Once Mencius met a man who was going to try to prevent a war by explaining to the two kings involved how unprofitable it would be for them. The idealistic Mencius praised the man's purpose but advised him that this reasoning would lead the ministers, officers, and soldiers of the countries to act from the motivation of personal gain, and a state where such considerations of profit prevailed would be bound to be ruined. However, if he were to convince them with humanity and righteousness, and the people were to learn to act out of the goodness of their hearts, then that state would become a true kingdom. Such a state would surely have the Mandate of Heaven. Mencius once said, "He who with a large state serves a small one conforms to Heaven. He who with a small state serves a large one stands in awe of Heaven. He who conforms to Heaven preserves the world, while he who stands in awe of Heaven preserves his own state."

King Hsiang of Liang asked Mencius how the world may be at peace: Mencius advised him, "When there is unity, there will be peace." When the king asked who could unify the world, Mencius replied that if there was one man among the "shepherds of men" who did not delight in killing men, then all the people would look to him and gladly follow. Like Confucius, Mencius rejected high taxes and warfare; he said, "Those who are skillful in warfare deserve the severest punishment." To Mencius the military experts are the great criminals. "If the sovereign of a state loves humanity, he will have no enemy in the world." The sage achieves humane government by means of education not by means of weapons of war. Mencius cites the expedition of King Wu: "The king said, 'Fear not! Let me bring peace to you. I am not making war against the people.' On hearing this, the people bowed their heads and prostrated themselves to the ground. 'To battle' is to rectify. Everyone wishing himself to be rectified, what need is there for war?"

Indian Mystics: Mahavira and the Buddha

"Hatred does not cease by hatred at any time,
but hatred ceases by love;
this is an eternal truth."

Buddha

"Peace to all beings."

Buddhist greeting

The *Upanishads* of the seventh and sixth centuries B.C. are mystical writings of the seers *(rishis)* of ancient India who practiced yoga to attain conscious union with God. They taught that the soul *(atman)* is the same essence as God *(Brahma),* eternal and immortal. The soul incarnates in the world of appearance or illusion and is responsible for the consequences of its actions *(karma).* The soul continues to reincarnate until the consciousness re-awakens to its inherent divinity and is liberated from the wheel of rebirth. The knowledge that the true self *(atman)* is a part of God is a psychological liberation, and the awareness of one's own immortality frees one from the fear of death and brings a feeling of eternal peace. As the Jews often use the word for peace *(shalom)* as a greeting, the Hindus often conclude their prayers with peace *(shanti).* The *Maitri Upanishad* describes the way of meditating on sound by which one ascends to non-sound resulting in complete union and also peacefulness. India has a long tradition of its mystics who renounce the world and go off to find internal peace and liberation. In a transcendental sense it is believed that if one person finds eternal peace and spiritual liberation the entire world is spiritually benefited.

One such person was Nataputta Vardhamana (599-527 B.C.) who was given the name Mahavira which means "Great Hero." As the historical reformer of the Jain religion, the Jains believe Mahavira to be the twenty-fourth and last of the great teachers. Mahavira made *ahimsa* the essential principle of the religion. *Ahimsa* has been translated as "non-violence," but it literally means not hurting or not harming. Mahavira was the younger son of a local king and was brought up amidst luxury. He married and had a daughter. After his parents died of voluntary starvation, at the age of thirty he gained his older brother's consent (after a year of waiting for it) to leave the palace, give away all his possessions, and retire from the world. He joined a monastery, limited himself to one garment, and pulled out his hair in five handfuls. The *Akaranga Sutra* describes his discipline: "Neglecting his body, the venerable ascetic Mahavira meditated on his soul, in blameless lodgings, in blameless wandering, in restraint, kindness, avoidance of sinful influence, chaste life, in patience, freedom from passion, contentment; control, circumspectness, practicing religious postures and acts; walking the path of nirvana and liberation, which is the fruit of good conduct. Living thus he with equanimity bore, endured, sustained, and suffered all calamities arising from divine powers, men, and animals, with undisturbed and unafflicted mind, careful of body, speech, and mind." After a few months he threw away the robe and left the monastery to wander naked through the plains and villages of central India. Not wanting to become attached to any place or person he never stayed more than one day in a village or more than five days in a city, except during the rainy season when he did not want to tread on paths that were teeming with life. He took asceticism and *ahimsa* to their extreme limits. He completely disregarded his body, staying in the cold winter shade and the hot summer sun; even when people physically beat him he paid no attention. He was extraordinarily careful not to injure any form of life while walking or sitting. He strained the water he drank and ate only left-over food that had been prepared for others and had no germinating life in it. After twelve years of practicing these austerities he became liberated and free of all attachment to the world. Then he taught others for thirty years before he passed out of the world. He emphasized the five great vows: 1) *ahimsa* or non-killing and non-injury, 2) non-lying or speaking only the truth, 3) non-taking or not stealing or being greedy in even its subtlest forms, 4) celibacy and renunciation of all sensual pleasures, and 5) non-attachment or not being delighted or disturbed by any outward experience. These disciplines were later incorporated into the preliminary step of Patanjali's *Yoga Sutras,* the classical text of yoga.

Certainly one cannot expect everyone to become as ascetic as the extreme Mahavira, but he demonstrated its effectiveness. *Ahimsa* is a cardinal principle in the way of peace, and non-injury is well supported by the self-disciplines which control lying, stealing, greed, lust, and attachment. For people to be at peace with each other, such self-restraint is essential.

Gautama Siddartha (563-483 B.C.) was also born as a prince in a small state in India. To prevent him from renouncing the world his father surrounded him with every luxury and removed all signs of old age, disease, death, and religious men. Gautama married and spent his time in the pleasure gardens of the palace. However, by providence the prince happened to observe on his way to the pleasure garden first an old man, then a sick man, a corpse being carried to a funeral, and finally a begging monk. Never having witnessed such sights before, Gautama began to seriously contemplate the meaning of life and its inevitable decay, suffering and death; like the monk he too must try to find a solution to these problems. Therefore he escaped from the palace and became an ascetic, as Mahavira had done. He gave up everything he had in order to beg for his food and search for enlightenment. For six years he tried to mortify the flesh. Not bothering to wash, the dirt fell off of him in cakes. Fasting and eating only one seed a day he became so thin that he could grab his spinal column from the front. Finally he collapsed and was near death, but it was at this point that he realized that practicing extreme austerities was not the way to enlightenment and liberation. He had already gained five disciples; but when he went back to begging for food, they all left him. Gautama concentrated on meditation; while sitting under the Bo tree, he overcame all temptations and entered into nirvana or supreme peace. People did not know what to make of this person and inquired whether he was a god, a devil, an angel, a man, or what. Gautama replied simply, "I am awake." Thus he became known as the Buddha, which means the awakened one or the enlightened one.

Buddha based his teaching on four noble truths: 1) that life is painful and suffering, 2) that desire and attachment are what causes the pain and suffering, 3) that pain and suffering may be eliminated by ceasing to desire and be attached to things, and 4)

12

that the way to eliminate the pain and suffering is by means of the eightfold path which is right understanding, right purpose, right speech, right action, right livelihood, right effort, right concentration, and right meditation. Having experienced both the extremes of luxury and asceticism, Buddha discovered that the middle way between them was the easiest path. His common sense and acute psychological insights into the whole process of consciousness and its tendencies toward bondage enabled the Buddha to teach a universal doctrine which would work for many people. His middle path was easily accessible to everyone, and he encouraged women as well as men to follow his path of enlightenment. He demonstrated and taught what he called the fourfold infinite mind of love, compassion, rejoicing, and equanimity.

For fifty years he taught, and his following grew steadily. One year when there had been a drought, a dispute developed between the Sakyas and the Koliyas over the water of the Rohini River. As the conflict increased to the brink of war, the Buddha placed himself on the river bank and asked why the Sakya and Koliya princes had assembled. They replied that they were about to do battle, and he asked why. The princes were not sure, so they asked the commanders who had to ask the regent who in turn questioned the farmers on the details. The Buddha then asked them to compare the value of the water and the earth to the value of the princes and men. After a while the Buddha was able to persuade them to refrain from fighting, and thus much bloodshed was avoided.

The Buddha taught that one ought to give ungrudging love even to the man who foolishly does wrong to one. Such a man hearing this about the Buddha went to him and abused him. The Buddha silently pitied his folly. When the man finished, the Buddha asked him to whom a present would belong if a person refused to accept it. The man replied that it would still belong to the one who offered it. The Buddha then told the man that he could keep his abuse, and he observed what a misery it would be for the man. The Buddha said to him, "A wicked man who reproaches a virtuous one is like one who looks up and spits at heaven; the spittle soils not the heaven, but comes back and defiles his own person. The slanderer is like one who flings dust at another when the wind is contrary; the dust does but return on him who threw it. The virtuous man cannot be hurt, and the misery that the other would inflict comes back on himself." The abusing man was ashamed and later became a follower of the Buddha.

Even when Devadatta, one of the disciples, tried to have the Buddha murdered because he had not been chosen as his successor, the Buddha harbored no resentment. The hired assassins were converted by the Buddha's loving kindness. When Devadatta caused a schism in the order, the Buddha allowed everyone to follow whomever they chose. Finally when Devadatta was dying and suffering the torment of his own karma, the Buddha assisted him spiritually so that in a future incarnation he would have a good opportunity to attain Buddhahood.

The ethical teachings of the Buddha are poetically expressed in the *Dhammapada.* What we are is the result of our thoughts. The person who is always complaining is full of hatred, while the person who forgives is filled with love. "Everyone trembles at punishment, everyone loves life; remember that you are like them, and do not kill nor cause slaughter." Do not speak harshly to anyone, for angry speech is painful. "Let a person overcome anger by love, let him overcome evil by good; let him overcome greed by generosity, and lying by truth." The person who uses violence is not just; rather the just person learns and uses intelligence to distinguish right from wrong and to guide others. A good person is tolerant with the intolerant, mild with the violent, and free from greed among the greedy.

In the third century B.C. the great King Ashoka was converted to Buddhism and promoted Buddhist teachings throughout India and even sent Buddhist teachers to the rulers of Syria, Egypt, Cyrene, Macedonia, and Epirus. He financed Buddhist education and erected pillars in many places declaring his intention to practice and spread the *dharma* (doctrine, duty). No longer would he conquer by arms and punishments, but he would be merciful and encourage devotion. He ruled the tremendous domain of most of India and portions of Afghanistan, Sind,

Kashmir, Nepal, and the lower Himalaya. During his reign there were protected wells, public granaries, medical treatment for all people and even for animals, and public servants to prevent unjust imprisonment and to help large families and the aged. Animals, birds, and forests were protected, and King Ashoka became a vegetarian and lived like a Buddhist monk even while he ruled the greatest empire of his time.

Early in the Christian era Buddhism spread to China and from there to Japan and also Tibet. The Buddhist way of life has been a tremendous influence toward peace and has been the most dominant religion of the Orient.

3
Greek Conscience: Pythagoras, Socrates, and Aristophanes

"Don't stir the fire with a knife."

Pythagoras

"Let no man by word or deed persuade you
To do or to say that which is not best for you."

Pythagoras

"I myself would wish neither;
but if it were necessary either to do wrong or to suffer it,
I should choose to suffer rather than to do wrong."

Socrates

"O that Love would you and me unite in endless harmony."

Aristophanes

Pythagoras lived during that sixth century B.C. which gave so many inspired religious leaders to mankind. He was born in Samos and studied with Pherecydes who was considered one of the seven sages of ancient Greece. He traveled widely and visited Epimenides and the cave of Ida on the island of Crete. He was initiated into the mysteries of Greece and those of the Chaldaeans and Magi. He entered the sacred temples of Egypt, learned the Egyptian language, and gained the secret spiritual knowledge from the priests. When he returned to his homeland of Samos, he found it under the tyranny of Polycrates. So he went to Crotona in Italy where he developed a constitution for the city and started his mystery school which soon had about three hundred students.

Pythagoras claimed that he could remember his previous incarnations. His school taught both exoteric and esoteric doctrines. After a preliminary period of silently listening to him speak in the dark, students who passed certain tests of their spiritual commitment were allowed to enter the inner rooms and interact with Pythagoras. Exoterically Pythagoras developed the sciences of mathematics, geometry, and music. He taught that number is the law of the universe, while unity is the law of God. He discovered the mathematical relationships of the musical intervals and the famous theorem that in a right triangle the square on the hypotenuse is equal to the squares on the sides containing the right angle. He urged a simple life with a diet of uncooked fruits and vegetables and drinking only pure water as the best way to a healthy body and alert mind. He forbade the killing of animals. He believed that the soul is divine and immortal proceeding through a series of lifetimes, implying that evolution is the law of spiritual life. He taught that the seat of the soul extends from the heart to the brain and that the human psyche has three levels of consciousness — the instincts, emotion, and intelligence.

Most of the Pythagorean doctrines which became public were phrased in exoteric terms to protect the sacredness of the teachings from the profane. The inner meaning of some of his guidelines was explained by the classical writer Diogenes Laertius in his biography of Pythagoras.

Don't stir the fire with a knife: don't stir the passions or the swelling pride of the great (with violence). Don't step over the beam of a balance: don't overstep the bounds of equity and justice. Don't sit down on your bushel: have the same care of today and the future, a bushel being the day's ration. By not eating your heart he meant not wasting your life in troubles and pains. By saying do not turn around when you go abroad, he meant to advise those who are departing this life not to set their hearts' desire on living nor to be too much attracted by the pleasures of this life.

He encouraged people to behave in such a way that they would turn their enemies into friends rather than turning friends into enemies. Those in the school held their possessions in common, and he advised them to consider nothing their own. He warned people not to allow anyone to persuade them by words or action to do or say that which is not best for them, thus establishing the principle of individual conscience. He taught that man is akin to the divine and that God does care about man. For Pythagoras the most important thing in human life is the art of winning the soul to good. Virtue, health, all good and God are harmonious, and therefore all things are constructed according to the laws of harmony. Friendship is harmony and equality.

Late in life Pythagoras married Theano and had a daughter Damo and a son Telauges. Pythagoras found himself in the middle of a conflict when there was a revolution in Sybaris and five hundred refugees came to Crotona for sanctuary. The Sybarites demanded them back, which would have meant certain death for them. Having granted them political asylum the Pythagoreans refused to give them up, and a battle resulted in which Sybaris was destroyed.

Pythagorean teachings were quite influential in classical Greece. Empedocles who lived in the fifth century B.C. studied Pythagorean doctrine with Telauges, the son of Pythagoras. When Empedocles published his poetry and made the teachings public, the Pythagoreans decided to exclude poets. Later on Plato was also excommunicated for revealing the esoteric doctrinés.

Empedocles considered himself a god and it was said that he performed healings, prophecies, and miracles. He taught that there are two principles in the universe — Love and Strife — and that everyone is always following one or the other. The Golden Age is when people are following the law of love, friendship, and concord. In the Golden Age love is even extended to animals, and all of life coexists in peace and harmony. He also believed that the soul is divine and immortal and that it may spend many lifetimes following Strife until the rule of Love is learned. Empedocles cried out, "Will you not cease from ill-sounding bloodshed? Don't you see that in careless folly you are consuming each other?" Since mankind is one family, it is like a father slaughtering his son and like children eating the flesh of their parents.

Greek religion from at least the time of Hesiod had a divinity called Peace *(Irene),* and in this cult animal sacrifices were not allowed. Peace was depicted in sculpture as the mother of Wealth *(Plutus).* Many of the religious cults of ancient Greece joined together in amphictyonic leagues in order to preserve peace by means of mediation and conciliation between the city states. They protected people and sacred places by maintaining neutrality in time of war. They had a religious authority, but the council was composed of representatives from the various cities, giving it a democratic or federalist structure as a confederation of states. The most important amphictyonic council was Delphi which served the Greek peninsula. The Ionians of Asia Minor were in the Delian amphictyony. The Delphic council exercised judicial powers and could be used to arbitrate disagreements. Even when wars did break out amphictyonic law prohibited member states from cutting off water supplies and burning down cities; those who disobeyed these rules were liable to be destroyed by total war.

Socrates (469-399 B.C.) took the cue for his life-long search for wisdom from the Delphic oracle which declared that there was no one wiser than Socrates. Socrates tried to find someone who was wiser, but came to realize that God alone is wise and that the oracle had recognized him for knowing this truth. Socrates was a great teacher although he never claimed to be such nor did he accept money for his conversation. He spent his entire life in the city of Athens except when he served as a citizen soldier on the military expeditions to Potidaea, Amphipolis, and Delium. He was praised for his courage by the general Laches after he fought off foes during their retreat at Delium, and Alcibiades said that Socrates saved his life at Potidaea and then encouraged the generals to give the prize of valor to the officer Alcibiades rather than himself. Obviously Socrates was not a pacifist, but he stands out for his zealous love of justice and obedience to his own conscience. He struggled for justice as a private citizen, because he felt that if he had become a public statesman he would probably have been put to death even sooner. However, when his tribe was serving as Prytanes it became his duty to preside over the Athenian Senate. This assembly attempted to put on trial together the naval commanders who had not buried the dead after their victory at Arginusae. Socrates believed that this was clearly illegal — first to group them together, second not to allow them time to prepare their defense, and third because the popular assembly was not a court and had no right to condemn to death. Socrates went against strong popular opinion of the time and flatly refused to support the illegality. Even though orators threatened to impeach and arrest him, Socrates decided that it would be better for him to run the risk for the sake of the law and justice rather than participate in the injustice out of fear of imprisonment and death. The six men were condemned and executed, even though the illegality was generally recognized afterwards. This occurred under a democratic government. During the oligarchical government of the Thirty Socrates was summoned and ordered with four other men to bring in Leon from Salamis to be put to death. Socrates later explained that these commands were given to people in order to implicate as many as possible in their crimes. Socrates again risked death rather than do something unjust or unholy, as even the strong arm of that oppressive government could not frighten him into doing wrong. Although the other four men went to Salamis and fetched Leon, Socrates went directly home; and he might have forfeited his life if that government had not been shortly thrown out of power.

Finally Socrates was put to death by those who resented his criticisms and feared his spiritual influence on others, particularly the youth. He would not agree to stop his pursuit of wisdom and justice as he saw them, and in his trial he courted death and was given that sentence. Although given an opportunity to escape from prison, Socrates chose to obey the law — even though in this case it meant his own execution — rather than to run away like a coward. The first well-known martyr of recorded history, Socrates positively worked for good and did not resist with any form of violence the evil threats and actions taken against him.

Socrates often discussed justice and how the ideal state would operate both for the individual and in society. He counters the traditional idea that we ought to help our friends and harm our enemies by showing that justice never does wrong or harm; therefore to be just we must not harm anyone. Since justice is a virtue of balance, health, and harmony, and since virtue leads to true happiness, then it is wise for us to be just. Justice is good and healthy for the individual soul and for society, while injustice is a spiritual cancer for both. Only one thing is worse than committing wrong and that is to fail to correct the wrong. Thus Socrates implies that we not only ought to refrain from unjust actions, but that it is also essential to the health of our society that we work to correct any injustices that may be occurring. In addition to his personal example the way that Socrates endeavored to do this was by educating people to follow justice above all. In his conversations he continually worked to bring more awareness to the other speakers on whatever topic was being discussed. Yet he always allowed them their freedom of choice as he assisted them in looking at new viewpoints. In Plato's *Republic* which is supposed to describe the ideal state there is a key turning point in the discussion where Socrates and the others disagree on the best state, and Socrates willingly follows Glaucon and others who wish to create a "luxurious" state. Socrates had suggested a simple life-style which would be harmonious and peaceful, but it soon becomes clear that a state which wants more than it is able to produce and fairly trade for will have to take over the land and goods of its neighbors. Such a luxurious and feverish state must be prepared for war and maintain a strong military force. Certianly such a military state which takes advantage of other states by force of arms is suffering from the disease of injustice, and the use of resources to support the army makes it even worse. Yet Socrates clearly pinpointed that the origin of such an imperialist state can be found in the greed of its citizens who desire more than their fair share of the goods the world is able to produce. The terrible irony is that the misdirection of human resources into the military reduces the amount of constructive goods and increases the suffering from destructive conflicts between states. Tragically the heroic battles that the Greeks fought in self-defense against the Persian invasions of 490 and 480 B.C. were later followed by the Peloponnesian War between the Greek city states of Athens and Sparta and their respective allies.

Aristophanes wrote several comedies criticizing and satirizing the Peloponnesian War which lasted from 431 to 404 B.C. In his earliest play which is still extant, *The Acharnians* (425 B.C.), Dikaiopolis (which means "just city") is an Athenian farmer who had to leave his land to find refuge in the city. He manages to get a private treaty with Sparta which frees him from military service. He criticizes the Athenians for rejecting the peace proposals with Sparta. He is accused of treason by the Acharnian charcoal burners, but escapes by borrowing a costume from Euripides. Dikaiopolis cleverly manages to have a feast amid the poverty.

In the following year Aristophanes produced *The Knights* in which he satirized Cleon, the most powerful politician in Athens. After *The Acharnians* had been presented, Cleon brought charges against Aristophanes in the Public Assembly and in the Courts saying that he had "slandered the city in the presence of foreigners." In *The Knights* Cleon is held up to ridicule as 'the Paphlagonian' and 'the Tanner.' The Athenians were so terrified of Cleon that no artist would make a mask to represent him and no actor would play the part. Therefore Aristophanes put on ruddy make-up and played the role himself. In the play the Paphlagonian is put down through his own methods of flattery, boasting, and invective by the Sausage-seller. Although the play was received enthusiastically and won first prize, Cleon remained in favor.

In *The Peace* Trygaeus flies up to heaven on a great dung-beetle and discusses peace and war with Hermes. War is shown mixing a salad from various cities in a gigantic mortar. Aristophanes points out how ambitious military officers and weapons merchants prolong war, and then he describes how peace brings blessings to people:

"You can leave your darts behind you:
    yea, for sword and spear shall cease.
All things all around are teeming
    with the mellow gifts of Peace."

Finally Trygaeaus returns to earth with the companions of Peace: Harvesthome and Mayfair. Aristophanes shows how the crest-maker, breastplate-seller, trumpeter, helmet-seller, and spear-burnisher will all be put out of business.

The most famous of the anti-war plays is *Lysistrata* (411 B.C.) in which the lady of that name organizes the women of Athens and Sparta to go on strike until a peace treaty is concluded. Lysistrata gets the women to take a vow to refrain from willingly granting any sexual favors to their husbands. The women take over the state treasury at the Acropolis. To speed the plot along the wives and mistresses adorn themselves in transparent gowns to seduce the men. The men of Athens and Sparta become sexually aroused and not being granted any satisfaction they impatiently arrange a hasty peace treaty. The play is a poignant and ribald representation of the power of women to correct the follies of an aggressive masculine world by making a choice of the popular slogan — "Make love not war."

4
Jesus and the Early Christians

"Blessed are the peacemakers,
for they shall be called the children of God."

Jesus

"But I tell you: love your enemies,
do good to those who hate you,
bless those cursing you, pray for those abusing you,
so that you may become sons of your Father in heaven."

Jesus

"Shall it be held lawful to make an occupation of the sword,
when the Lord proclaimed that he who takes the sword
shall also perish by the sword?"

Tertullian

"For we no longer take up 'sword against nation'
nor do we 'learn war any more,'
having become children of peace,
for the sake of Jesus, who is our leader."

Origen

Probably the greatest exemplar and teacher of peace is Jesus the Christ. Jesus has been considered by many to be the fulfillment of the Jewish prophecies concerning the coming of a Messiah, the Prince of Peace. His birth as well as his death was shrouded in miracle, myth, and tragedy. Angels were said to have greeted his mother with the blessing of "peace on earth." Persian magi (astrologer-priests) found their way to the child by cosmic guidance, and Herod fearing the birth of a rival king had innocent babies slaughtered in Bethlehem. Jesus, however, escaped to Egypt. Little was recorded about his childhood and youth, but it is likely that he may have studied with teachers in Egypt, Persia , and India. At the age of twelve he was debating with rabbis in Jerusalem. Suddenly in his thirties he appeared at the Jordan River to be baptized by John. After fasting in the desert he began to preach and call his disciples. When his messianic attitude was challenged in the synagogue at Nazareth he had to escape from a violent mob. He traveled throughout

Israel healing the crippled, the blind, the deaf, lepers, and the psychotic (demonized) while preaching his message of love and forgiveness to the common people. His extraordinary abilities included reviving the dead and manifesting food for thousands. On one of these occasions the people wanted to make him their king, but he escaped from this crowd also.

Finally he entered Jerusalem triumphantly and taught in the temple during Passover week. In his zeal to reform the Jewish religion he aggressively overturned the money-changers' tables, freed the pigeons and doves which were being sold for sacrifice, and criticized the hypocrisy of the Pharisees and Sadducees. Figuring he was a revolutionary against the Romans as well, the resentful priests tried to trap him by asking whether the Jews should pay taxes to Caesar. In his wisdom Jesus replied that the coins with Caesar's image may be returned to the material power but the spiritual aspects of life are to be devoted to God. Although Jesus had no worldly authority or power, his spiritual power was so great that it was changing people's consciousness rapidly. Afraid of this threat to the status quo the leaders of the Jews and Romans combined together to arrest him, try him, and execute him by crucifixion. Jesus knew that this would take place, but he submitted to it to fulfill the divine will and demonstrate a faith which transcends physical death. His personal will faced this test in the garden at Gethsemane. At one point he advised the disciples to get a couple of swords, perhaps so that they would feel safe and protected when he was taken; for he did not want anyone to suffer except himself. When Judas Iscariot brought the soldiers to arrest him, Peter cut off the ear of a servant; but Jesus immediately halted the violence, saying, "No more of this! Put the sword into the sheath; for all who take a sword will die by a sword." Jesus then healed the servant's ear as he pointed out how he could have called forth thousands of angels but that it was not God's will to interfere in that way. He took care to see that his disciples were allowed to go free. During his trial Jesus indicated that his kingdom was beyond the physical world, and therefore his followers do not fight. He did not resist the violence inflicted upon him, and he did not compromise the truth as he knew it. Even while nails were being driven into his body, he forgave those who were acting out of ignorance. The purity of his love in the face of mockery, torture, and death, along with his miraculous ability to bring the body back to life again makes this the most famous and influential event in the history of mankind.

Jesus taught the spiritual life of love, mercy, forgiveness, and charity. He declared that those who really care about justice and making peace are blessed by God. Those who are kind and gentle and pure in heart are the ones living in the kingdom of heaven; even when they are persecuted while working for justice, it is a blessing because it is transmuting the negativity of the persecutors and purging the world. Going beyond the karmic law of Moses he taught that we can enter the grace of God by forgiving each other's mistakes and correcting our ways. He went deeper than just outward action to indicate an inner morality which leads to peace of mind and heart. Not only is killing wrong, but even to be angry toward a brother can upset this inner peace. Therefore it is better to talk to the person and come to an understanding so that our love can flow. It is not our place to strike back or to punish others, for these actions tend to perpetuate ill feelings and conflict. Therefore Jesus recommended that we not resist evil, for by fighting one who does evil we would fall into that negative game and increase the violence. By not resisting the negativity of others it can be released and dissolved most easily; our responsibility is to keep ourselves free of negativity. Traditionally people tried to love their neighbors and hate their enemies, but to achieve spiritual oneness we must love our enemies. By doing good even to those who hate and abuse us we become like God who loves all. Thus loving everyone unconditionally is a way to realize God; also this love tends to dissolve the hatred and conflicts.

Jesus maintained a peaceful consciousness and advised others to live in peace. "Go in peace," he would say, and he counseled his disciples to go out and minister greeting people by saying, "Peace to this house." They were to look for a person of peace to stay with, and if they did not find one he advised them to let their peace return to them. However, Jesus was not satisfied with the common coin of what people think of as peace in this world. He

26

did not come to pacify people in their ignorance. In lifting people into spiritual consciousness some conflicts are inevitable, and his teachings certainly stimulated arguments and disagreements and divisions, often within a family. Each person must choose, and a conflict of ideas can be creative without being harmful to anyone.

When entering Jerusalem Jesus lamented that the people did not know the things that were needed to bring peace. He could foresee the problems and in fact predicted the destruction of Jerusalem which occurred in 70 A.D. Seeing the pattern of human civilization he also prophesied that just before the Christ consciousness becomes widely realized there would be wars, rumors of wars, and revolutions as nations are raised against nations. Earthquakes, plagues, and famines will be the birth pangs of the new age. Many people will point out individuals and claim they are Christs, but eventually the Christ will manifest and become apparent to everyone. Mystically Jesus gave his peace to his disciples, and in a transcendental way offers this peace to anyone who will follow his way. In the Christ consciousness one may find peace.

After the crucifixion and resurrection the organization of the Christians began to grow. They were persecuted by Jews (including Saul of Tarsus who became Paul), and some, like Stephen, even sacrificed their lives as they testified to their faith in Christ. Led by Peter and a converted Paul the cult increased and spread throughout the Roman world by peaceful means even in the face of violent persecution. The faith of the martyrs influenced many conversions, and the loving fellowship was attractive to many. As the religion became stronger it rivaled the authority of the Roman state. Many Christians had to choose whether or not to serve in the Roman army and obey the Roman cults which deified the emperor. About 200 A.D. Tertullian wrote in defense of a Christian soldier who had refused to wear a certain crown because he regarded it as a pagan act in conflict with his faith. Tertullian questions whether warfare and military service is proper for Christians. How can a son of peace engage in battle, torture, and punishment when he has been advised by Christ not to sue at law or avenge his own wrongs? Tertullian recommended that Christians serve Christ rather than the militia of the emperor. He believed that war was the most evil of all earthly activities and ought to be avoided in every case.

Origen was the son of Christian parents, and his father was martyred in 203. He applied philosophy to Biblical scholarship; he taught reincarnation and refused to believe in everlasting damnation. He became a priest in Alexandria where he was head of a school, but he was deposed by Bishop Demetrius. He found refuge in Palestine where he taught for nineteen years. During the Decian persecutions (249-251 A.D.) he was imprisoned and tortured, and he died four years later.

Origen wrote, "There is peace when no one lives in a state of discord, when no one gives way to quarrelsomeness and there is no hostility or cruelty." He felt that the earth is so infested with war that peace could be achieved only by God's grace and that this would amaze even the angels. His most famous essay was a rebuttal to Celsus who had accused Christianity of undermining the Roman state, particularly by Christians' refusal to perform military service. However, Origen took the position that the Christians could convert even the barbarians to justice and humility by their peaceful methods. The unity of mankind must go beyond the Roman empire of the pagans' concept to include everyone in the whole world. Christians, he felt, owed their allegiance to Christ above the emperor, and they could not take up arms for any cause, although they could pray for the empire.

An example of the Christian-Roman conflict over military service was the case of Maximilian, a twenty-year-old Numidian, who was called to be enrolled as a soldier in 295 A.D. He declared, "I am a Christian, and cannot fight." The proconsul Dion tried to mark him, but he refused. Dion gave him the choice: "Bear arms, or you shall die." Maximilian asserted that he was not a soldier of this world, but a soldier of God. Dion asked him who persuaded him, and he said that it was his own mind and the one who called him. Dion tried to get his father to convince him, but the father said his son knew what was best for him. Maximilian continued to refuse to bear arms. Even when he was told that other Christians are soldiers and fight, he replied, "They know best what is expedient for them; but I am a Christian, and it is unlawful to do evil." Believing that he was going to Christ, Maximilian was beheaded.

When the Emperor Constantine was converted to Christianity in 313, Christianity became established as the religion of the Roman Empire, and the views of Christians on war and military service changed radically. Only the Donatists in North Africa remained pacifists in the face of "Christian" Roman militarism, and they were condemned for it.

There was an incident during the reign of the last pagan Roman Emperor Julian involving Saint Martin, the founder of probably the first monastery in the West. Martin had reluctantly become a Roman soldier at age fifteen. He took the occasion to seek discharge when Julian was presenting the soldiers individually with a donative. Martin asserted that he had served Caesar as a soldier but that now he was a soldier of Christ and would not fight. Julian called him a coward who was afraid of battle, but Martin declared that he would march unarmed into the ranks of the enemy protected by the cross. He was ordered into prison, and he was determined to prove his words. However, on the next day the enemy sued for peace and surrendered.

5
St. Francis of Assisi and the Magna Charta

"Where there is charity and wisdom,
there is neither fear nor ignorance.
Where there is patience and humility,
there is neither anger nor vexation.
Where there is poverty and joy,
there is neither greed nor avarice.
Where there is peace and meditation,
there is neither anxiety nor doubt."

Francis of Assisi

"No freeman shall be taken, nor imprisoned, nor disseized,
nor outlawed, nor exiled, nor destroyed in any manner;
nor will we pass upon him, nor condemn him,
but by the lawful judgment of his peers,
or by the law of the land.
We will sell to none,
we will deny nor delay to none right and justice."

Magna Charta

Francis of Assisi (1182-1226) was the son of a rich cloth merchant. He was born while his father was traveling in France; his mother named him John, after the beloved disciple, but when his father returned he changed his name to Francis, for the country which had enthralled him. When he was twenty the Perugians made war on Assisi, and Francis was imprisoned for a year with some of the nobles from his city. Francis dreamed of becoming a knight and winning glory. While he was delirious with sickness, a voice asked him why he left the Lord to serve a vassal. He decided to renounce military glory, and he returned to Assisi where he began to serve the sick and the poor and to rebuild three churches in the area.

Following the teachings of the Christ as closely as possible he and his disciples vowed to live in abject poverty while doing works of Christian charity. Within eleven years there were over five thousand Franciscan Friars. He also founded the Poor

Clares for women and later the Third Order for people who lived in the world. The Rules of the Franciscan Order were ratified by Pope Innocent III. In 1210 the preaching of Francis led to an agreement between the upper and lower classes of Assisi which foreshadowed the Magna Charta by granting bondsmen the right to free themselves from their lords.

During the Crusade of 1212 he gained permission from the Pope to be an unarmed standard-bearer of Christ; he sailed for Syria, but a storm cancelled the journey in Slavonia. The next year he decided to carry the Gospel to Morocco; this time serious illness forced Francis to return to Italy again. Finally in 1219 Francis made it to Egypt. He preached reform in a Christian camp, and then in spite of warnings of the danger he entered Saracen territory. When he and his companion were seized and bound, Francis shouted, "Sultan! Sultan!" Brought to the Sultan he shared the message of Christ and challenged a priest of Mohammed to enter the flames with him to see whose faith was stronger. The Sultan was impressed by his courage and gave Francis gold, silver, silk, and precious things, but Francis refused them all. The Sultan let the two friars go free and gave Francis and his fellows permission to travel through Saracen lands; whereupon Francis visited Bethlehem, Jerusalem and Mount Calvary. In the last year of his life Francis, though ill, helped to make peace between the Bishop and the podesta who were feuding in Assisi. He composed new verses for his Sun Song:

> Praised be thou, O Lord,
> for those who give pardon for thy love
> and endure infirmity and tribulation,
> blessed those, who endure in peace,
> who will be, Most High, crowned by thee!

Following the song the podesta and Bishop Guido embraced and forgave each other.

A most symbolic legend of St. Francis is how he tamed the fierce wolf who was ravaging the city of Gubbio. Francis encountered the wolf with the sign of the cross and then explained to the animal the wrongs he had done in devouring beasts and killing people. In bringing peace to the wolf Francis promised that the people of Gubbio would feed him so that hunger would no longer drive him to these crimes. The wolf obediently followed Francis, and the citizens were amazed. Francis then preached to the people how they ought to give up their fear and take care of the wolf by providing food, which they all agreed to do. Many other stories also reveal how Francis loved all of God's creatures.

Once Brother Leo asked Francis what perfect joy is. Francis related that if, they, when wet, cold, and muddy, knocked on a convent door, and the porter refused to let them in but drove them away like a couple of thieves, beating them with clubs until they nearly died, "and if we endure all this so patiently, and think of the sufferings of Christ, the All-praised One, and of how much we ought to suffer for the sake of our love of him — O Brother Leo, mark thou, that in this is perfect joy." Perhaps the teachings of Francis are best conveyed by the simple prayer which he lived so well.

> Lord, make me an instrument of Thy peace:
> Where there is hatred, let me sow love;
> Where there is injury, pardon;
> Where there is discord, union;
> Where there is doubt, faith;
> Where there is despair, hope;
> Where there is darkness, light!
> O Divine Master, grant that I may not so much seek
> To be consoled, as to console;
> To be understood, as to understand;
> To be loved, as to love;
> For it is in giving that we receive,
> It is in pardoning that we are pardoned,
> And it is in dying that we are born to Eternal Life.

From 1199 to 1216 King John caused tremendous turmoil in his attempts to rule England. One of the results of his ineptness was the signing of the Great Charter (Magna Charta). The prime mover behind this great breakthrough in human rights was a man named Stephen Langton. By oppressing the provinces of Anjou, Touraine, Maine, and Normandy, John lost the support of their barons, and after some battles these provinces were taken over by King Philip of France. Although Pope Innocent III had assisted John against Philip, John's refusal to grant the payments due from Richard's will led to a quarrel with the Pope over the appointment of a new Archbishop of Canterbury. The younger monks of Canterbury had selected and installed Reginald, immediately sending him off to Rome to be confirmed by the Pope. John, who frequently acted out of anger and resentment, demanded that the Bishop of Norwich, John de Grey, be elected instead, and the King sent off a deputation to the Pope with a gift of twelve thousand marks. Pope Innocent III responded to all of this by choosing his own man, Stephen Langton. Stephen was born in England and had become the leading teacher at the university in Paris. He agreed with Becket's view that the lordship of God was higher than the power of kings. In Paris Stephen taught Lothario who at the age of 37 became Pope Innocent III. The new Pope called his friend to Rome where Stephen became the most popular preacher. Stephen was a biblical scholar and helped future generations by dividing the Scriptures into chapters. He also wrote histories of Henry II and Richard and composed the hymn, *Veni, Sancte Spiritus,* which is sung in England as *Come, Thou Holy Spirit, Come.* The Pope released John's representatives from their promise to him, and eleven of the twelve canons were won over to Innocent's choice of the capable Stephen.

John, however, refused to allow Stephen Langton to enter England, and the Pope retaliated by pronouncing an interdict on John's domain, which closed the churches and cancelled all religious services and rituals. John started confiscating church property, and Innocent excommunicated the King. As a diversion John fought battles in Ireland, Scotland, and Wales, but the lack of religious rituals to which they were so accustomed must have deeply affected the people. Meanwhile Stephen resided at Pontigny, studied the situation, and wrote letters to the important people in England; it was made a criminal offense to read these letters. Finally the king invited Cardinal Langton to meet him at Dover, but Stephen refused because he had been addressed as cardinal instead of archbishop. He asked John to pay for everything the Church had lost. In 1212 the Pope freed all subjects of John from their oaths of allegiance to him and declared that anyone who served the King was excommunicated. The Pope then deposed John and granted his crown to Philip. The French prepared to invade England, but the English, afraid for their own safety, rallied their defenses. Although the English were winning a naval battle at the time, John was afraid and made an agreement with the papal legate Pandulf to return ecclesiastical property, submit his crown to the Pope in feudal vassalage, and pay an annual tribute for the withdrawal of the decrees of interdict, excommunication, and deposition. John thus ruled England as a papal fief, and churchmen were reinstated. Langton was received by a prostrated John, but the Archbishop could not give him the kiss of peace because the ban of excommunication was still in effect. In Winchester Cathedral Stephen did absolve John of his sins and perform the Holy Eucharist, although Innocent resented this infringement of his prerogative. Innocent had to call off Philip who was prepared for war, and the French King was so frustrated that he attacked Flanders.

Finally after another year the interdict was lifted. John attacked France to try to win back the lost provinces, but he had little support from the English aristocracy who felt that they had been sold out to Rome. While John was away, Stephen Langton preached at St. Paul's in London and held a meeting with the barons in which he produced an old document signed by Henry I which granted specific English liberties. When John returned defeated from France, he tried to take out his animosity by demanding scutage or payment from all who had not supported military service. The barons, stimulated by Stephen's research and ideas, demanded a return to these laws certified by Henry I. They gathered their forces which outnumbered the King's and met John at Runnymede. Stephen Langton with the help of Saire de Quincey spent four days drafting a document that everyone could accept. This Great Charter which was signed there on June 15, 1215 has been considered perhaps the most important document in English history. They agreed upon liberties and principles of law which could protect people from the tyrannical actions of men in power. The rights of habeas corpus, due process of law, and trial by jury were formulated. Although no implementation procedures were instituted, it became a standard to which everyone could refer, and the idea of a parliamentary council was included.

John immediately tried to renounce the agreement by appealing to the Pope. The ailing Innocent annulled the Charter and excommunicated the barons. However, Stephen Langton refused to publish the edict and left for Rome, while church authorities suspended the Archbishop for two years and helped John raise an army of mercenaries. At Rome Langton was castigated by the Pope and was not allowed to speak at the Fourth Lateran Council when he was denounced and the barons were condemned as disobedient vassals. This same council, which determined to fight a crusade against the Cathari, Waldenses, and Albigenses (which were the most peace-loving sects in medieval Christianity), confirmed the suspension of Stephen Langton as Archbishop of Canterbury. Stephen thought of becoming a Carthusian monk, but stood by helplessly as the church forced England into a civil war. King John's mercenaries defeated the barons who asked for the help of France's King Louis. Louis was excommunicated for invading England; his French forces and the barons could only hold London against John. However, both John and Innocent III died, and the English nobles were reconciled with Henry III and his regent so that Louis had to return to France. After all this folly the Charter remained, and in the reign of Edward I Parliament was developed.

6
Dante on One Government and Chaucer on Counseling Peace

"It is in the quietude or tranquility of peace that mankind finds the best conditions for fulfilling its proper task."

Dante

"The human race is at its best when most free."

Dante

*"For Solomon says that
when the condition of a man is pleasant and to God's liking,
He changes the hearts of that man's enemies
and constrains them to seek peace of him, and grace."*

Chaucer

Efforts to establish peace throughout Europe began in the tenth century as the French Church organized a peace movement in various places and persuaded nobles to renounce and outlaw private war and violence in order to protect pilgrims and travelers. In 989 a council at Charroux, France, declared the *Pax Dei* (Peace of God) which prohibited men from forcing their way into churches to plunder them and from usurping the property of peasants. Anyone using violence on noncombatants in war was to be excommunicated. In 1023 in a conference at Mouzon, Robert the Pious of France and Emperor Henry II discussed the idea of a universal peace pact for France and Germany and eventually for all Christendom. Starting in 1027 the Truce of God was proclaimed, and in the twelfth century it became part of civil and canon law. Armistices were used to stop feuding parties; bishops got people to take pledges for peace; and private wars were suspended during Lent,, harvest season, and from Wednesday evening to Monday morning of each week. The German Henry III, son of Henry II, cooperated with the Truce of God, and at Constance in 1043 he pardoned all those who had injured him and encouraged his subjects to renounce vengeance and hatred. The decision to launch the Crusades by Pope Urban II in 1095 may have been partially prompted by a desire to remove the warlike elements from Europe by bringing the Christians together and sending them off to fight the Moslems.

Gerohus of Regensburg made a proposal to abolish war during the Third Crusade in 1190. He suggested that the Pope forbid all war and that any conflicts between princes be decided by arbitration in Rome. Any ruler refusing to submit to the result of the arbitrating decision was to be excommunicated and deposed. The kings of the time were not ready to accept this policy, and as private wars lessened they became more involved in national wars; in the thirteenth century even the popes used war to serve their political purposes.

Pierre Dubois offered a plan for a league of nations in his book *The Recovery of the Holy Land* (1306). Dubois had studied at Paris under Thomas Aquinas and Siger de Brabant. He became a lawyer and was a member of the Estates General assembly. He was a chauvinist patriot who believed in a strong French military, and he wanted the French king to rule the West and East including Palestine and the Greek Empire. He suggested the education of both boys and girls for service in the East. He proposed that disputes between sovereign princes be settled by means of arbitration by a council of appointed clerics and laymen from each nation. He exhorted all Christian believers to join in peace and refrain from war, and he suggested as a penalty for violation the loss of property and exile to the Holy Land. Dubois wrote, "If it seems fitting to establish a league of universal peace in the manner prescribed, there should be a unanimous decision by the council of prelates and princes that all prelates of whatever rank, as well as secular knights owing service, shall solemnly swear to uphold with all their power this league of peace and its penalties, and in every possible way see that it is observed." Unfortunately his scheme was too biased in favor of the French.

Dante Alighieri was born at Florence under the sign of Gemini in 1265. He went to the Franciscan school of Santa Croce. As a young man he wrote romantic poetry *(New Life* 1292), and in 1295 he entered politics and served on the council. In 1300 he was elected as one of the six priors who ruled Florence. At the time Florence was rife with civic strife between two groups called the Whites and the Blacks. In his *History of Florence* Machiavelli mentions how Dante tried to make peace. "Both parties being in arms, the Signory, one of whom at that time was the poet Dante,

37

took courage, and from his advice and prudence, caused the people to rise for the preservation of order, and being joined by many from the country, they compelled the leaders of both parties to lay aside their arms, and banished Corso, with many of the Neri (Blacks)." Corso Donati was a relative of Dante's wife, and he had also agreed to banish his best friend, the poet Guido Cavalcanti, in his effort to be fair. Dante as a White opposed the interference of the Pope, but Pope Boniface VIII sent Charles of Valois to intervene. Charles helped the Blacks to power and exiled over six hundred Whites including Dante who was charged with corruption in office. While in exile Dante supported reconciliation and refused to take up arms against his native city of Florence even though he "formed a party by himself." In 1306 he was sent by Marchese Franceschino Malaspina as an ambassador to Sarzana where he concluded a peace with the Bishop of Luni. In 1310 when Henry VII set off for Rome with the Pope's approval to restore peace in Italy, Dante wrote a letter to the princes and people of Italy asking them to welcome Henry as a peacebringer. During this time Dante wrote his political treatise *Monarchy* in which he urged that everyone accept the Emperor as the temporal sovereign authority who could unite the world under one rule of law. Dante's masterpiece *Divina Commedia* was composed in exile and was completed shortly before he died in 1321 of a fever he caught while on a diplomatic mission.

Dante begins the treatise on one government with the idea that human beings with a divine nature who love truth ought to work for the benefit of future generations. Dante reasons that the function of mankind is to use the intellect both theoretically and practically in order to become fully actualized. He points out that the best conditions for fulfilling this purpose are tranquility and peace. "Hence it is clear that universal peace is the most excellent means of securing our happiness. This is why the message from on high to the shepherds announced neither wealth, nor pleasure, nor honor, nor long life, nor health, nor strength, nor beauty, but peace." Dante reasons that unity is best for humanity and assumes that unity would be achieved by having one ruler. This monarch would be the one to solve all disputes between princes.

Thus justice and order would be maintained. Dante shows how justice is lost because of personal desires, and again he assumes that the monarch will be least susceptible to these desires. However, Dante failed to realize the difficulties of having one person try to decide everything or delegate his authority. Dante states that mankind is best when it is most free, but he neglected the danger of tyranny from a single ruler. Nevertheless he did point the way to the unification of humanity under one rule of law and unanimous cooperation. He lamented the suffering of human strife and held out an idealistic vision of unity.

O humanity, in how many storms must you be tossed, how many shipwrecks must you endure, so long as you turn yourself into a many-headed beast lusting after a multiplicity of things! You are ailing in both your intellectual powers, as well as in heart: you pay no heed to the unshakable principles of your higher intellect, nor illumine your lower intellect with experience, nor tune your heart to the sweetness of divine counsel when it is breathed into you through the trumpet of the Holy Spirit: 'Behold how good and pleasant it is for brethren to dwell together in unity.'

Another great poet, Geoffrey Chaucer, served occasionally as a diplomat. When he was about twenty Chaucer was taken prisoner in France and ransomed by King Edward III. He then acted as a diplomatic courier in the negotiations that brought about the Peace of Calais in 1360. He married a lady of the English court and for ten years went on many diplomatic missions to France and the Low Countries "on the King's secret affairs." Chaucer was a close friend of John of Gaunt and was aided by him in court life. In 1372 he traveled to Florence and probably heard Boccacio's lectures on Dante, and in 1378 he went to Milan where Petrarch had spent his last twenty years. In 1385 Chaucer became justice of the peace for Kent, and the next year he was elected to parliament. He was given appointments by Richard II and was also favored by Henry IV; he died in 1400.

Chaucer is justly famous for his great work *The Canterbury Tales*. These stories told by various characters while on their pilgrimage to Thomas Becket's tomb illustrate many points of view on life from ribald accounts of lust to high moral fables. Each tale reveals the personality of the storyteller. Significantly, after he is cut off in his tale of a knight named Sir Thopas, the story that Chaucer puts into his own mouth is an enlightened account of peacemaking and diplomatic counseling called "The Tale of Melibeus."

Melibeus is a powerful and rich young man who has a wife named Prudence and a daughter Sophie. One day when Melibeus is out playing in the fields, three of his old enemies break into his house, beat his wife, and wound his daughter in five places. Melibeus becomes greatly upset and weeps profusely as Prudence attempts to console him. Melibeus decides to call in all the people he knows in order to get advice about what to do. Melibeus sadly describes his trouble and angrily speaks of vengeance and his eagerness for war. First the physicians help the wounded and declare their policy of never doing harm to anyone; however, they add that as diseases are cured by their opposite, so war might be cured by vengeance. Many flatterers praise the wealth and might of Melibeus and his friends while disparaging the strength of his enemies. The older and wiser recommend that he guard his person and his house, but that he wait before deciding on war. Then the young people rise up and begin to cry, "War, war!" An old man advises caution, but the young heckle him until he sits down. Melibeus is ready to go along with war when his wife Prudence asks him to listen to her counsel. Melibeus says he would be a fool to give over his sovereignty to a woman, women being evil and unable to keep secrets. Prudence declares that he ought to change if previous counsel has been foolish, that listening to advice is not giving up one's power to decide, and that all women are not necessarily bad and untrustworthy. Melibeus agrees to listen to Prudence.

First, she says, one ought to begin by praying to God for guidance. Then one must remove the three impediments to good counsel from the heart — anger, covetousness, and hastiness. After having taken counsel within oneself it is best to keep it secret so as to receive unprejudiced and objective counsel from the advisors. Melibeus had betrayed his desire, and all the flatterers had agreed with his passion. Prudence suggests that it is best to ask advice from friends that are old, faithful, discreet, and wise; he must beware of former enemies and those who are afraid of him.

Prudence teaches Melibeus that in counsel he ought to be truthful about the situation and examine the probable results of the advice and the various causes. Then Prudence takes up the specific issues. She points out that vengeance is not the opposite of wickedness as the physicians thought, but it is wrong for wrong; peace is the opposite of war. As to guarding his person and garrisoning his house, Prudence declares that friends are the best defense. War would be foolish because his enemies have more relatives than he and surely would revenge his acts of vengeance. Only a judge with the proper jurisdiction should punish. The consequences of war would be injuries, deaths, and the waste of wealth. Spiritually the ultimate cause of everything is God. Therefore if God has allowed this to happen to his family, it must be chastisement for previous sins. Allegorically the three enemies of mankind are the world, the flesh, and the devil, and the five wounds symbolize the five senses through which the sins have entered the heart. He should leave vengeance to the sovereign Judge, for " 'Vengeance is mine,' saith the Lord." Besides Melibeus does not have the power to avenge himself. Chaucer and Prudence discourage fighting under any circumstances: "It is madness in a man to strive with one who is stronger than himself; and to strive with a man of even strength is dangerous; but to strive with a weaker man is foolish. And for this reason a man should avoid all strife, in so far as he may."

Melibeus figures that he can count upon his wealth, but Prudence warns that no amount of wealth is sufficient to maintain war, and a great man is as easily killed in a war as a poor one. Prudence counsels Melibeus to make peace with God and become reconciled to His grace, and God will change the hearts of his enemies so that they also will seek peace. Prudence then tells the adversaries privately that they ought to repent for the injury and wrong they had done to Melibeus, herself, and her daughter. They are surprised by her gracious words and acknowledge the wrong they have done. She convinces them to

41

trust themselves to Melibeus and her for a reconciliation. She then gathers their true friends, and they being correctly informed give counsel for peace. When the adversaries submit, Melibeus still wants to punish them by confiscating all their property and banishing them, but Prudence warns him against gaining a reputation for covetousness and then advises mercy. Finally Melibeus forgives them for all the offenses, injuries, and wrongs done against his family so that God will forgive him the sins he has done in the world. Thus through Prudence Chaucer shows us how to alleviate the mood for war and bring reconciliation.

7
Erasmus and Humanism

"Peace is the highest good
to which even the lovers of the world
turn all their efforts."

Erasmus

"Our wars, for the most part,
proceed either from ambition, from anger and malice,
from the mere wantonness of unbridled power,
or from some other mental distemper."

Erasmus

"And so at last shall appear, how great madness it is,
with so great tumult, with so great labors,
with such intolerable expenses, with so many calamities,
affectionately to desire war:
whereas agreement might be bought with far less price."

Erasmus

Desiderius Erasmus was born on October 27, 1466 at Rotterdam; he was the second illegitimate son of a priest and a widow. He was educated by the Brethren of the Common Life who emphasized personal reform through Christian inwardness, though Erasmus later complained that they suppressed natural gifts by blows, reprimands, and severity. However, he was impressed with the classical learning by Alexander Hegius and the eminent humanist Rudolph Agricola. In 1484 both of his parents died, and Erasmus, who wanted to go to a university, was reluctantly lured into a monastic career by the promise of access to many books. Erasmus disliked monastic life, and seeking greater intellectual stimulation in 1492 he was ordained a priest and became secretary to the Bishop of Cambrai. He was given leave to attend the University of Paris for four years where he taught himself Greek and studied classics. However, just as the monastic rituals did not fulfill his deep spiritual longings neither did the scholastic theology and logic-chopping of Scotus and Ockham which he later satirized. Erasmus did not complete a degree in theology, but having tutored some Englishmen in Latin in 1499 one of them, William Blount, Lord Mountjoy, invited him to England for a year. There he met the humanists John Colet and Thomas More, and he began to study the early Fathers of the church for a more real and alive theology.

Erasmus lived and traveled in various places in Europe and became a great cosmopolitan man. His constitution was very sensitive, and he fled often from plagues and uncomfortable circumstances. He lived in the university city of Louvain, visited Renaissance Italy, spent several years in England, and resided for many years in the peaceful city of Basle. His first major work was a collection of classical quotations, *Adagia.* In 1503 Erasmus published his *Handbook of the Militant Christian* which laid down the principles for a spiritual Christian life.The book became quite popular and established his reputation. He exhorted Christians to be ever watchful and use the weapons of prayer and knowledge. The highest wisdom is to know yourself. We must learn to distinguish the inner man from the outer man. Erasmus wrote, "This then is the only road to happiness: first, know yourself; do not allow yourself to be led by the passions, but submit all things to the judgment of the reason . . . Nothing is harder than for a man to conquer himself, but there is no greater reward or blessing." Man is a combination of spirit and flesh. "The spirit has the capacity of making us divine; the flesh tends to bring out our animal nature." Spiritual love is not based on physical pleasure but is loving the Christ in another person. Erasmus listed guidelines for living a Christian life: have faith in the teachings of Christ; act in accordance with the teachings; analyze fears and dissolve them; make Christ the only goal; turn away from visible things to seek the invisible; love and follow Christ; stay free of vice; etc. He concluded the work with special remedies against lust, avarice, ambition, pride, and anger, about which he wrote:

> When resentment goads you to revenge, remember that anger is a false imitation of fortitude, and fortitude is the antithesis of anger. Nothing manifests a weaker will, nothing requires a feebler and weaker mind than enjoyment of revenge. In trying to appear brave by not allowing an

injury to go unpunished, a person displays only immaturity, since he cannot control his mind in a particular situation.

The most famous book of Erasmus, *The Praise of Folly,* was written in England and dedicated to Thomas More in 1511. The satire shows how popular and respected folly is among mankind and pokes fun at the foibles of the time. The church is not spared by Erasmus' caustic wit. Pope Julius II had recently led troops into battle. So Folly points out how the popes make war their only duty while morals are disregarded, and how this is hypocritical and contradicts Christ's teachings and principles.

In 1516 Erasmus published his new translation of *The New Testament* in Latin and also the *Education of a Christian Prince.* This latter work is in sharp contrast to the amorality of Machiavelli's *Prince* which was being written at this time. Erasmus advised current monarchs to maintain peace through justice, limit taxes to luxuries, and convert monasteries into schools. Erasmus encouraged all men and women to read the gospels and the writings of Paul, and his *New Testament* encouraged religious reform and paved the way for Luther who burst on the scene with his Theses in 1517. Erasmus supported many of Luther's reforms, but he was always wary of fanaticism and intolerance. He never really took sides between Luther and the Pope, although in 1524 he challenged Luther's theology by defending the freedom of the will. He cringed at peasants' rebellions and religious wars. The rest of his life Erasmus struggled in the face of criticism from both sides to plead for peace and tolerance of differences within the church. He advised Pope Adrian VI to refrain from punishing anyone and encouraged him to reform the abuses against which many had been crying out. Ill and upset by attacks made on him by Protestants and Catholics Erasmus finally died in 1536 without the sacraments of the Church but repeating the names of Mary and Christ.

Humanism was an intellectual and educational movement which began in Italy and spread throughout Europe in the fifteenth and sixteenth centuries. It was based on the discovery of classical literature and culture, and in liberalizing education it led to the Renaissance and the Reformation. Erasmus was probably the most influential humanist in northern Europe. In a time of religious fanaticism which was to continue for over a century Erasmus used his pen as a weapon for peace. As a humanist he always sought clarity and intelligent solutions to problems. He pointed out the futility and madness of war, especially for people who claim to be Christians. Even wild beasts do not murder each other in such large numbers over such trivial causes. How can those who are part of the unity in Christ war on each other? There is no real glory in war which injures people on both sides and causes such destruction. Human beings were given bodies designed for friendship not war; unlike other animals which have armor, horns, claws, tusks, prickles, poison, or speedy flight, humans are naked, weak, tender, with soft flesh and smooth skin. Furthermore the inward nature of man expresses reason, kindness, humor, tears, and speech. Erasmus asks if there is anything in the world better than friendship and love.

These ideas and others are expressed in a piece called *Against War*. Having described the original nature of man Erasmus contrasts this to the corrupted man of his time who slaughters other people and destroys towns. Man is supposed to be superior to other animals; yet beasts of the same species rarely fight each other; beasts kill or fight only from hunger or from self-preservation, and they use only natural weapons and armor; beasts usually fight alone and do not engage in mass violence. How has man degraded himself? Erasmus outlines the stages of man's development of war. The first use of violence was probably in self-defense against wild beasts, and this led to the hunting of dangerous animals and the custom of using their skins for winter clothing. In the second stage people gave up vegetarianism and began to gain pleasure from the cruel killing of animals as they became accustomed to flesh-eating. The habit of killing in the third stage led to occasional manslaughter. People began to praise those who punished "evildoers" by killing them. Men began to band together and use weapons. In the final stage empires developed and used offensive wars for greed and conquest. Tyrants made war their policy, and devious reasoning was employed to make the murder of strangers seem honorable. This for Erasmus was the contemporary situation. "War, what other thing is it than a common manslaughter of many men together, and a robbery, the which, the father it sprawls abroad, the more mischievous it is?"

What, then, can we do about it? Erasmus takes the position that even from self-interest war is extremely expensive and wasteful. If the leaders of both sides counted all the costs of a war, they would realize that it would be wiser to settle the disputes by arbitration. Even the worst natural disasters such as earthquakes, fires, floods, and plagues are not as bad as the man-made calamity of war. People have the use of reason to solve problems. Erasmus describes the suffering of the soldiers who must slaughter or be slaughtered. Neither is their material gain in war which must destroy towns before rebuilding them. The empire builders are really the enemies of mankind. Erasmus contrasts the peace of Christ and the early church to the frequent warfare of the Christians of his time. They try to justify themselves by scholastic sophistry and reference to civil laws. Erasmus refutes the six major arguments that had been used to rationalize a "just" war by Christian nations. Even if war was sanctioned by the *Old Testament,* Jews were not Christians, and Jesus ordered Peter to put up his sword. The use of both temporal and spiritual swords to war on heretics and infidels likewise was unjustifiable. The word of Christ himself has more authority than the theologians', even that of Thomas Aquinas. Punishing evildoers is not socially beneficial, because thousands of innocent people suffer in a war. Princes are not justified in fighting for their right, because they gain power only by the "consent of the people" who are "free by nature." People have the right to take their power back if the king abuses it by injuring the people. The traditional view that Christians can war against infidels like the Turks is hypocritical to the teachings of Christ and is hardly the way to convert anybody.

In *The Complaint of Peace* Erasmus pleads for peace by letting Peace speak. Peace laments that mankind has rejected the source of all their happiness, prosperity, and security. Peace observes the harmony and concord in the universe and how

47

elephants, sheep, cranes, jays, storks, dolphins, bees, and ants get along and work together. "Unanimity is of absolute necessity for man, yet neither nature, education, nor the rewards of concord and the disadvantages of disunity seem to be able to unite mankind in mutual love." Man's ability to speak and reason and cultivate friendship ought to lead to peace. Man benefits from reciprocity and mutual support, and thus cities have been constructed. Children depend upon parental care. Man is capable of peace, and the teaching of Christ is a powerful influence for peace; but somehow man has an insatiable desire for fighting, and dissension haunts the courts of princes. Peace turns to the scholars and philosophers, but here finds continual disputing. Even the monks are divided into factions. Peace hopes that in marriage concord might be found, but strife creeps in; even within individuals inclinations and reason struggle with each other. Yet the angels proclaimed peace on earth at the coming of Christ who also taught peace. The princes of this world put men in uniforms as a sign to whom they belong, but the Christ said that his disciples would be known only by the love they have for each other. Peace describes the love of Christ and peaceful qualities of true Christians. Mankind is one; all Christians are of the same religion, hope for the same salvation. "Christians should war against vice. Yet they ally themselves with vice to war against men. All pretense aside, ambitions, anger, and the desire for plunder are at the base of Christian wars." Peace is ashamed at the vain and superficial reasons which princes use to plunge the world into war. The desire for power is the most criminal of all causes of war. Peace complains that "Christians attack Christians with the very weapons of hell." Older and experienced leaders in government and in the church perpetrate war; thus a few cause the destruction of many. Peace asserts, "If they examined their consciences, they would find that the real reasons are anger, ambition, and stupidity." It is stupid, because they are not able to find a more intelligent solution. God is not deceived by the pretenses. Peace advises, "There are laws, learned men, pious abbotts, and reverend bishops whose mature counseling can bring these matters to a peaceful solution." Even if their arbitration decisions are not perfectly just, the result would be far superior to the ravages of war. Peace warns that confederations do not guarantee peace and often cause war.

We must look for peace by purging the very sources of war, false ambitions and evil desires. As long as individuals serve their own personal interests, the common good will suffer. No one achieves what he desires if the methods employed be evil. The princes should use their wisdom for the promotion of what is good for the entire populace.

The king should be like a father of a family and remember that the people are free citizens and fellow Christians, and the people ought to respect the king and support the common good. Consent and approval by the citizens is the check on the ambition of the prince. Those who work to secure peace and concord ought to be honored. There must be advisors to the ruler who are neither inexperienced so that they find war attractive nor in a position to profit by warfare. Peace concludes, "Nothing is more conducive to genuine peace than a sincere desire that comes from the heart." Every effort must be made to remove obstacles even though concessions must be made. Divisive hatreds and prejudices must be overcome. The costs of waging war must carefully be weighed – destruction of cities and fields, theft, murder, immorality, injury, and death, all at enormous expense. Finally Peace pleads with the princes, priests, theologians, and bishops to promote peace. Those who love peace must not allow the few who gain from war to have their way. In peace kingdoms will be ruled by law rather than by arms, the people will enjoy productivity and tranquility, and friendship and happiness will abound.

8

Crucé's Peace Plan and Grotius on International Law

"We must establish the reign of reason and justice,
and not violence, which is fit only for beasts."

Eméric Crucé

"After all, we are not looking for a hollow peace
nor for one lasting only three days,
but for one that will be voluntary, equal, and permanent,
a peace that will grant everyone what belongs to him:
full privileges to every citizen, hospitality to the stranger,
and freedom to travel and trade to everyone without exception."

Eméric Crucé

"For God has given conscience a judicial power
to be the sovereign guide of human actions,
by despising whose admonitions
the mind is stupified into brutal hardness."

Hugo Grotius

Eméric Crucé (1590-1648) was a monk who taught at a *collège* in Paris. He was a classical scholar little known except for his treatise on universal peace entitled *The New Cineas* which was published in 1623 with a second edition in 1624. This work is the first practical proposal for world peace which does not aggrandize the power of a particular nation, empire, or religion. Crucé declares in the preface that "No one can say that he has strayed from the path of truth out of love either for his country or his religion, even though these loves are so engraved on his soul that death itself cannot efface them." He wrote during the early years of the Thirty Years' War, and his ideas probably influenced the Peace of Westphalia in 1648. His concept of a universal and perpetual peace was adopted by the Duke of Sully in his description of Henry IV's "Grand Design" (for this idea did not appear in the 1620 edition of Sully's work but was fully treated in the 1638 edition), and also Hugo Grotius would have known of it when he was in Paris writing *The Rights of War and Peace* (for he was a close friend of Crucé's rival Gronovius). In an age of religious intolerance and fanatical wars over conflicts in theology and church ritual, Crucé put forward a tolerant and universal vision of peace and justice. He states in the preface, "I know that heresies must be refuted, but I see none greater than the error made by those who place injustice above all else and who value only arms."

Not only was Crucé the first to suggest a political solution whose primary aim was world peace, but he also was the first to consider the economic implications and goals, which his subtitle indicates: "Discourse on Opportunities and Means for Establishing a General Peace and Freedom of Trade Throughout the World." He addresses himself to the current monarchs and sovereign rulers, and clearly his method is to reason with them and institute his program from the top down. Crucé claims that he will show them ways to make their states secure through establishing universal peace which is in the public interest, and he begs them to have pity on the human race and stop the abuses of horrible wars. Crucé points out four main causes of war: honor, profit, righting some wrong, and exercise; religion, he says, "usually serves as a mere pretext." Crucé criticizes the common opinion that the exercise of arms is noble and glorious. "Ordinary valor" is brute force, but magnanimity and steadfast courage make for true valor which is "to reject all wrongs and to do none." Actually there is more dishonor than honor to be found in war — insults and scorn to prisoners and ignominious death. Princes ought to be ashamed of warmongering and curtail their ambition. As for profit, more often than not the costs of war are tremendously expensive even for the winning side. The avenging of past wrongs is precarious, because sovereigns rule by the grace of God and too often their attempts to fight for what they think they have a right to does not meet with God's providence; many kingdoms have been lost by rulers who tried to exterminate some other power they believed to be unjust. Long possession indicates God's favor, and therefore conquest is not just. Instead of resorting to arms to settle disputes, they ought to submit their cases to arbitration by sovereign rulers not involved in the particular case. The danger of war due to restless activity requires several remedies. First the sovereigns must maintain control of their armies and not let the militarists take over. Princes ought to be proud of maintaining peace and justice rather than trying to

51

aggrandize themselves through conquest. Games and hunting can exercise and release the tensions of the more aggressive. With universal peace agreed upon the army can be greatly reduced, while at the same time bona fide police and peace officers can be paid larger wages. Manpower can be put to work in agriculture, trade, and in building needed canals. Pirates and enemies can be given opportunities to work through public assistance programs. Artists and craftsmen can be encouraged by offering rewards for excellent work.

Religious conflicts can be overcome by realizing "the basic similarity in men's nature which is the true foundation of friendship and human society." Ultimately all religions have the same goal of adoration of God which is found in the heart. True piety does not lead to animosity, malice, hostility, and slander. "One must be a good man and have charity, without which faith is useless. Anyone lacking this virtue does not have religion engraven in his heart." Crucé warns against the arrogance of trying to correct others' beliefs by force. Wrong actions may be punished by civil laws, but only God who sees men's hearts and their secret thoughts can judge questions of understanding. The Emperor Charles V had attempted to suppress Lutheranism in its beginnings, but was forced by his new enemy to grant them freedom of conscience in order to preserve his own state.

Crucé proposed that there be an assembly of ambassadors from every nation in the world including Tartary, Persia, China, Ethiopia, and the East and West Indies. He suggested Venice as the meeting place, because it was neutral, central, and accessible. Decisions were to be made by the whole assembly which could easily bring violators "back to the path of reason." Laws would be passed by the majority of votes and would be enforced with arms. Princes must remain within their established boundaries and must not go beyond them for any reason. Complaints could be presented to the general assembly which would decide them. Crucé declares that the peace would be extremely valuable to all the monarchs.

Then Crucé turns to the means necessary to maintain the domestic peace within each country. The monarch must govern moderately according to reason and with care for all the people.

Vice and crimes must be justly punished, and the ruler must be especially careful to root out flatterers and financial schemers from his own court. Rewards of honor and profit may be used to encourage good works. The poor must be provided for, and if they are healthy they may be taught trades. Crucé is quite critical of lawyers and legal tricks and formalities which delay justice and make it expensive. He recommends judges of integrity and simplification of legal suits and processes. Taxes which are necessary to the state ought to be based on land and the ability to pay, and trade ought to be universal without restrictions between nations. Public grain ought to be stored up in case of famine. Crucé encourages lawful recreation such as athletics, theatre, and music. The power of censure ought to be used to regulate morals and by the influence of public opinion keep people upright. Those who lead dissolute lives may lose their privileges — a senator his position, a knight his title, a citizen his civic rights. Crucé recommends education for the young which includes reading, writing, arithemetic, history and laws, languages, and exercise.

Between states the borders are to be kept the same, trade may be arranged, and foreigners must be treated justly. Weights, measures, and money must be standardized to prevent cheating. Crucé concludes with a description of the horrors of war which are caused by the sins of arrogance and cruelty. With little provocation thousands of men clash with each other, resulting in slaughter, dismemberment, and misery. Then innocent people are massacred, women violated, temples profaned. Famine and pestilence follow. Crucé exhorts us to renounce arrogance and cruelty so that wars will cease.

Huig de Groot, known by the Latin form Hugo Grotius, was born in Delft, Holland on April 10, 1583. His father was a burgomaster and Curator of the University of Leyden. By the age of eight Hugo was writing Latin poetry, and at twelve he entered the University and studied under the great scholar Joseph Scaliger. At fifteen he left the University, and serving the statesman Barneveld he traveled on a diplomatic mission to France where Henry IV called him "The Miracle of Holland." In

1600 he was admitted to the bar and settled at The Hague to practice law with Barneveld and the Dutch East India merchants. He married in 1609, and became official historian of the United Provinces and advocate-general of Holland and Zeeland. In his book *Mare Liberum* he challenged the claims of England, Spain, and Portugal to rule over portions of the ocean. He argued that the liberty of the sea is essential to the right of nations to communicate with each other and that no nation can monopolize ocean highways because of the immensity of the sea and its lack of stability and fixed limits. In 1613 he was appointed to the high legal office Pensionary of Rotterdam and went to England on a diplomatic mission concerning the freedom of the sea. Speaking for a group in his country Grotius urged King James to convene an international council to work on reuniting the divided Christian Churches.

In Holland again Grotius became involved in the Arminian controversy under the leadership of Barneveld in a political struggle against the Calvinists. He took the side of free will against the theory of predestination. Grotius wrote a passionate appeal in support of the Edict of Pacification which recommended tolerance. However, Maurice, the political leader, allied himself with the church and fanatical peasants against the Edict of Pacification. Representing the States of Holland Grotius publicly addressed the authorities of Amsterdam in favor of tolerating the two theological opinions; considering the political danger to the country and the religious danger to Protestantism, he pleaded for toleration and peace. But these were intolerant times, and his address was treated with contempt and suppressed by force. Though his family and friends advised him to give up the struggle, he devised a new formula for peace to be signed by both parties which did not contradict Calvinism and proposed a council to settle the question peacefully. This also was rejected by the fanatics and Maurice.

In 1619 Barneveld and Grotius were arrested as conspirators against the state; Barneveld was executed, and Grotius was sentenced to life imprisonment. His wife was allowed to join him, and he was provided with writing materials and books. However, in 1621 his wife concealed him in a chest for books, and he escaped to Paris where his wife later joined him. He then wrote a letter to the Netherlands authorities declaring that no one had been bribed to aid his escape, that he did not consider himself guilty of any crime against his country, and that nothing had happened to cause him to love his country any less. Barely surviving on a small and irregular pension from Louis XIII, Grotius began in 1623 his great work, *De Jure Belli ac Pacis (The Rights of War and Peace),* which was published in 1625. The Catholic Church proscribed the work in the index in 1627. The influence of the work spread though, as the Thirty Years' War was in midstream. The monarch of Sweden, Gustavus Adolphus, kept a copy of it next to his Bible under his soldier's pillow during the campaigns of the war. He commended Grotius before his death on the battlefield in 1633, and Grotius was selected as an ambassador of Sweden to negotiate a new alliance with France. Preoccupied with writing religious dramas and poetry Grotius was put off by Cardinal Richelieu's arrogance, and they quarreled over precedence and court etiquette. One of his books, *Truth of Christianity,* was enormously popular among Catholics and various Protestant sects, because it focused on the essential teachings of Christianity rather than the sectarian questions which divided Christians. This Latin book was translated into French five times, into German three times, and into English, Swedish, Danish, Flemish, Greek, Chinese, Malay, Persian, and Arabic. In 1645 he returned to Sweden where Queen Christina, who liked to patronize scholars and philosophers, tried to retain him. However, he decided to go home; his ship was caught in a storm, and he fell ill and finally died at Rostock on August 28, 1645.

Although he believed that there could be a "just war" (unlike Erasmus and other pacifists), Grotius made a tremendous contribution toward international law and a more just and moral conduct during wars. Living during an age of cruel and lawless religious and national warfare, *The Rights of War and Peace* delineated codes of justice for protecting innocent non-combatants, discerning rights of persons and property, and arranging methods for truces, treaties, and humane treatment of hostages and prisoners. In the Prolegomena Grotius asserts the need for these principles. "I saw in the whole Christian world a license of fighting at which even barbarous nations might blush. Wars were begun on trifling pretexts or none at all, and carried on without any reverence for law, Divine or human. A declaration of war seemed to let loose every crime." Although he often quoted scripture, Grotius derived his principles using human reason from the Law of Nature and the Law of Nations which are universally accepted. A civil right derives from the laws of a sovereign state, "But the law of nations is a more extensive right, deriving its authority from the consent of all, or at least of many nations." Wars over religion cannot be justified, because religion is a question of conscience and inner conviction which cannot be forced on anyone. Therefore wars against infidel nations or heretics are unjust, and no law can make a belief or disbelief a crime. Especially in doubtful cases we must listen to our conscience which can guide human actions in accordance with justice and reason. He quotes Cicero: "There are two ways of ending a dispute, discussion and force; the latter manner is simply that of brute beasts, the former is proper to human beings gifted with reason: men are obliged then to recur to violence only when reason fails." Grotius discusses three methods that can be used to settle disputes peacefully. The first is conference and negotiation between the two adversaries. The second he calls compromise, which is when a third party arbitrates the conflict and arranges a solution. The third method is to decide by lot or single combat. Grotius advises that it is often better to relinquish a right than to try to enforce it. In arbitration he emphasizes that it is important to choose a just judge who has integrity.

9

George Fox, William Penn and Friends

"All Friends everywhere, this I charge you,
which is the word of the Lord God unto you all,
Live in peace, in Christ, the way of peace,
and therein seek the peace of all men, and no man's hurt . . .
It is love that overcomes
and not hatred with hatred, nor strife with strife.
Therefore live all in the peaceable life,
doing good to all men."

George Fox

"We have suffered all along
because we would not take up carnal weapons
to fight withal against any,
and are thus made a prey upon
because we are the innocent lambs of Christ
and cannot avengê ourselves.
These things are left upon your hearts to consider."

George Fox

"I deplore two principles in religion,
obedience upon authority without conviction
and destroying them that differ with me for Christ's sake."

William Penn

"Peace is maintained by justice,
which is a fruit of government,
as government is from society,
and society from consent."

William Penn

George Fox was born in a small hamlet in Leicestershire, England in July, 1624. His father was a weaver and a pious warden of the church. George had little education other than learning to read and write and study the Bible. He was apprenticed to a shoemaker for whom he also tended sheep. In an incident at the age of 19 George was disgusted by tavern companions who tried to get him into a drinking match. That night he had a vision from God, and the next day, November 9,

1643, he left his family and trade to wander in search of true religion. Carrying his Bible he slept in fields or stayed with hospitable families. He questioned priests and argued with them. George searched for people he called "tender" who were loving and spiritually open. He discovered that most of the priests were not open but that many of the Seekers, a new sect, were. George Fox experienced "openings" or revelations which told him that both Catholics and Protestants could be sincere Christians, that universities like Oxford and Cambridge bred vain and deceitful priests, and that God did not dwell in church buildings as much as in people's hearts. Fox called the man-made temples "steeple-houses" and considered the church to be the community of believers in its original sense. Although he considered the Bible a valuable reference point, the inner Light takes precedence as the direct guidance of the Holy Spirit. Fox declared that revelation had not ended, but the insights from within must be checked to see that they are in harmony with the teachings of the Bible. There was the danger that some would be led astray by spirits of darkness or the devil; therefore someone attuned to the inner Light must discern the difference, and George Fox always felt that he could.

Fox had a powerful personality and an inner conviction which he would not compromise. Confident that the word of God was speaking through him he challenged priests and interrupted their sermons. He would speak for hours at a time, and sometimes he would just glare at people for as long as two or three hours. He could outshout just about anybody. He criticized social injustices, such as the hiring fair at Mansfield in 1648 where local justices had fixed a maximum wage for farm labor. He believed in human equality and was firm in practicing it, even in seemingly trivial ways. He would refuse to remove his hat before a judge or a king. Following the admonition of Jesus in the Sermon on the Mount he refused to take oaths. Because of these behaviors and his frank speech he was arrested many times. Altogether in his life he spent seven years in jail, often in filthy conditions, which he sought to reform. As Jesus called his disciples friends, so Fox referred to those who followed the inner Light as Friends, but the world gave them the name Quakers. Critical of professional priests, Fox believed that each person could relate to God directly and thus minister. He defended the rights of women to equal spirituality even against the views of other Friends. Fox and his followers were continually persecuted and often arrested for refusing to take oaths or for holding unauthorized religious meetings. Fox and other missionaries traveled to Europe and America to convince others of the truth of the inner Light. In America Fox preached to the Indians whom he treated as equals, and he urged humane treatment of Negroes and their eventual release from enslavement.

Following the teachings of the Christ closely, Fox was a pacifist, and the Society of Friends to this day has remained perhaps the most important pacifist religion. In 1651 during the civil war when Fox was in jail, some commissioners and soldiers offered to make him a captain over the soldiers who were eager to be led by such a courageous man. However, Fox told them that he "lived in the virtue of that life and power that took away the occasion of all wars," and he explained that all wars come from lust, as James pointed out in the Bible. When they realized that his refusal was serious, they threw him into a dungeon for almost six months "amongst thirty felons in a lousy, stinking low place in the ground without any bed." Thereupon Fox took to writing letters to judges against the death penalty for stealing and minor offenses, and he urged speedier trials because many were being corrupted by criminals in jails while they were waiting for their trials to begin. Then a Justice Bennet offered him press-money if he would be a soldier, but again Fox declined.

While preaching he warned soldiers not to do violence to any man. In March 1655 Fox wrote a letter to Oliver Cromwell, the Lord Protector, clarifying his pacifist position as "the son of God who is sent to stand a witness against all violence and against all the works of darkness, and to turn people from the darkness to the light, and to bring them from the occasion of the war and from the occasion of the magistrate's sword." He also referred to "the light in all your consciences, which makes no covenant with death, to which light in you all I speak, and am clear." Fox exhorted all Friends to live in peace; he declared that those who use carnal weapons throw away spiritual weapons, and those who do not love one another and love enemies are out of Christ's doctrine.

With the Restoration of a monarch in 1660 George Fox was again arrested without good reason. He wrote a letter to Charles II telling the King that he was the very opposite of a disturber of the peace. The suspicion that he would plot an armed rebellion was absurd. He asserted that he loved everyone including his enemies and attempted to awaken the love of the King for the truth. "Those that follow Christ in the spirit, the captain of their salvation, deny the carnal weapons." While in custody of soldiers at Whitehall he preached the gospel of loving one another and asked them why they wore swords and when they would "break them to pieces and come to the gospel of peace." Later that year Fox and eleven others signed "A Declaration from the harmless and innocent people of God, called Quakers, against all plotters and fighters in the world." They stated that their principle is, and their practices always have been, to seek peace and follow righteousness and the knowledge of God for the welfare of all. Warfare results from the lust and desire to have men's lives and estates. Pertinent passages from the Bible are quoted, but more importantly they honestly can declare that they have practiced the ways of peace and suffered persecution for righteousness' sake and have not done violence against anyone. They have suffered in obedience to God, having been "Despised, beaten, stoned, wounded, stocked, whipped, imprisoned, haled out of synagogues, cast into dungeons and noisome vaults where many have died in bonds, shut up from our friends, denied needful sustenance for many days together, with other the like cruelties." Hundreds of Friends had suffered these things, few more than George Fox. Yet they refused to swear or to fight; often they remained in jail after their sentence, because they refused to pay the jailkeeper since they did not recognize that they had committed a crime. They pleaded to the King so that he would end this useless suffering. In his *Journal* Fox described how this declaration cleared away the darkness so that the King proclaimed that no soldiers should search a house without a constable and that Friends in jail should be set at liberty without having to pay the fees. Fox continued to preach and clarify the doctrines of the inner Light until he died in 1691; during all this time he was the generally acknowledged leader of the Quakers.

The second great Quaker leader, William Penn, was born in London on October 14, 1644 and died in 1718. His father rose to become Vice Admiral of England and was knighted by Charles II. He was hopeful that his son would become prominent in the court and provided him with a fine education. Young William studied at Christ's Church College in Oxford where John Locke was teaching, but he was fined and expelled for refusing to attend church and for religious noncomformity. Disgruntled by his son's pious seriousness, the Admiral sent him off to France, and the father was glad when William returned a good French scholar with the bearing of the courtly life. He advised William then to study law at Lincoln's Inn, but after a year a great plague hit London in 1665. Again William turned toward religion and was convinced by a Quaker named Thomas Loe when he spoke about "a faith that overcomes the world." William recalled how the Lord had appeared to him since the age of twelve, the debauchery of Oxford and his persecution there, and the "irreligiousness" of the world's religions. At the Quaker meeting the Lord visited him again, and he testified, "I related the bitter mockings and scornings that fell upon me, the displeasure of my parents, the cruelty and invective of the priests, the strangeness of all my companions, and what a sign and wonder they made of me; but, above all, that great cross of resisting and watching against my own vain affections and thoughts."

A year later Penn was arrested at a meeting of Friends; the mayor, noticing his aristocratic dress, offered to free him on his promise to behave, but the twenty-three-year-old refused and was sent to prison with the eighteen others. Penn wrote, "Religion, which is at once my crime and mine innocence, makes me a prisoner to a mayor's malice, but mine own free man." In this letter to the Earl of Orrery he pleaded for religious toleration. The arrest brought the conflict between William and his father to a head. His father wanted him to conform to the ways of the world and attain a position of honor, but William pleaded that he must listen to his conscience. Finally his father threatened to disinherit him; he asked that his son only uncover his head before the king, the duke, and himself. William prayed and fasted to know the heavenly will; but this only strengthened his resolution, and he was thrown out of the house.

Uncertain about whether to give up his fine clothes, it is said that Penn asked George Fox if he must stop wearing a sword. Fox replied, "Wear it as long as thou canst." Penn gave up the sword and became an active promoter of Quaker ideas by writing numerous pamphlets such as "No Cross, No Crown," "The Great Case of Liberty of Conscience Debated," "Examination of Liberty Spiritual," "A Persuasive to Moderation," "The Rise and Progress of the People called Quakers," "Primitive Christianity Revived," etc. Many Quakers believed that his writings brought about the release of thirteen hundred Quakers from jail. Penn himself had been arrested again for preaching in 1670 because of the Conventicle Act. Penn challenged the legality of the indictment; when the magistrates did not like the jury's verdict, they locked up the jury without meat, drink, fire, and tobacco waiting for "a verdict such as the Court will accept." Penn referred to the rights of the Magna Charta and advised the jurors, "Give not away your right." The result was that Penn and all twelve of the jury were sent to prison. This trial became famous and showed that the arbitrary and oppressive proceedings of the courts badly needed reform. Again the next year he was sent to Newgate prison for six months for preaching without taking an oath, even though the law was only for those in holy orders, which Penn was not. He occupied the time in prison writing.

When Penn's father died, he gave his son his blessing. The crown of England owed a great debt of gratitude to Admiral Penn, and in 1680 William Penn asked for a grant of American land west of the Delaware. The land he received, probably the largest piece of property ever owned by a commoner, became the scene of the Holy Experiment in pacifist government and was called Pennsylvania. Penn wanted to call it Sylvania for its forests, but the King insisted that Penn be added. Although Penn was sole proprietor and therefore governor, he wanted it to be a haven for religious toleration and representative government. Of course it was to be a home for the Quakers, but others were welcome also. He drew up a constitution, and the first article protected freedom of worship according to conscience. Penn was sensitive to being friendly and peaceful toward the Indians and required that all land bought from him must also be purchased from the local tribes. In 1682 he gave the following address to the American Indians:

> The Great Spirit who made me and you, who rules the heavens and the earth, and who knows the innermost thoughts of men, knows that I and my friends have a hearty desire to live in peace and friendship with you, and to serve you to the utmost of our power. It is not our custom to use hostile weapons against our fellow creatures, for which reason we have come unarmed. Our object is not to do injury, and thus provoke the Great Spirit, but to do good.
> We are met on the broad pathway of good faith and goodwill, so that no advantage is to be taken on either side, but all to be openness, brotherhood, and love.

Penn stayed in America for two years overseeing the founding of the city of brotherly love, Philadelphia, and when he returned to England he was pleased to report that there was "not one soldier, or arms borne, or militia man seen, since I was first in Pennsylvania." Penn had to spend most of his time in England trying to protect the colony from intrusions by the British government; he was only to make one more two-year trip to Pennsylvania. He appointed deputies and encouraged the province to be self-governing. Although often barely a majority, Quakers tended to control the policies and were able to refrain from military activities and policies until 1756, in spite of frequent outside pressures to tax for defense or raise a militia. Although the Holy Experiment was not totally successful, it did demonstrate that a pacifist government could sustain itself even on a frontier with a vastly different type of people (Indians).

In 1693 William Penn published one of the world's excellent plans for international peace entitled "An Essay towards the Present and Future Peace of Europe By the Establishment of an European Diet, Parliament, or Estates." His points are relatively simple and well argued. First, the value of peace is obvious when we look at the terrible ravages of wars which cause so much suffering and destruction. Second, war and strife are prevented by means of justice, both for individuals and groups, resolving conflicts in a fair way. Third, justice depends on government to enforce laws impartially, and government gains its sovereign authority to do so from the consent of the people. Fourth, peace in Europe may be maintained by forming a Sovereign Parliament of the European states to collectively decide disputes and unite as one strength in enforcing the decisions. Fifth, there are three ways the peace is broken: defending one's own territory, trying to recover territory previously claimed, and trying to increase one's dominion by invading another country. Sixth, governments claim sovereignty by succession, election, marriage, purchase, or conquest. Seventh, all of the European states including Russia and Turkey should be included in the Diet with votes equivalent to the value of their territory. Eighth, among regulations a secret ballot is recommended to prevent the corruption of bribes with the idea that the one bribing would have no guarantee whether his money was effective. In the ninth section Penn answers objections. Even if the strongest nation refused to join, the others together could compel it. Small forces within each country could prevent a large army from forming. Youth not trained for war would not become effeminant if they were disciplined for some other type of work. States would still maintain their sovereignty over their own internal affairs. In the tenth section Penn lists the many benefits of his plan. Bloodshed would be prevented, and towns and property would not be destroyed. The Christian countries would be more in harmony with the true teachings of Christ. Every country would save money which could be used in more constructive ways. It would give the Christian countries security against the Turks. Travel between states would be free and easy, and personal friendships could develop between the peoples of different countries. Princes would not have to marry for political and diplomatic reasons but could establish unions based on sincere love. In his conclusion Penn reiterates the important principle that there must be a sovereign authority to settle disputes which is greater than the parties in conflict. Just as individuals have difficulty settling their own disagreements, so also nations often require an impartial authority to decide between them. As an actual example of a working federal system he cites the United Provinces which met at The Hague. Many of the principles of Penn's plan are certainly of lasting value.

10
Federalist Peace Plans of Rousseau, Bentham, and Kant

"Conscience is the voice of the soul."

Jean-Jacques Rousseau

*"Firmly convinced as I am that nothing on this earth
is worth purchase at the price of human blood,
and that there is no more liberty anywhere
than in the heart of the just man,
I feel, however, that it is natural for people of courage,
who were born free,
to prefer an honorable death to dull servitude."*

Jean-Jacques Rousseau

*"All trade is in its essence advantageous —
even to that party to whom it is least so.
All war is in its essence ruinous;
and yet the great employments of government
are to treasure up occasions of war,
and to put fetters upon trade."*

Jeremy Bentham

*"When the worst comes to the worst,
peace may always be had by some unessential sacrifice."*

Jeremy Bentham

*"If only freedom is granted, enlightenment is almost sure to
follow."*

Immanuel Kant

"Dare to know! Have courage to use your own reason!"

Immanuel Kant

*"Reason, from its throne of supreme legislating authority,
absolutely condemns war as a legal recourse
and makes a state of peace a direct duty,
even though peace cannot be established or secured
except by a compact among nations."*

Immanuel Kant

Jean-Jacques Rousseau was a fascinating individual whose unorthodox ideas and passionate prose caused a flurry of interest in 18th century France, and his republican sentiments for liberty, equality, and brotherhood led eventually to the French Revolution. He was born on June 28, 1712, but his mother died in giving birth to him. His father had him reading romances and classical histories such as Plutarch before apprenticing him to an engraver. Rousseau loved to walk in nature; frustrated at being locked outside the city gates of Geneva at nightfall, at the age of sixteen he left his home to wander on his own. He was guided by a Catholic priest to Madame de Warens who took him in for about ten years and eventually became his mistress. Rousseau studied music and devised a new system of musical notation which was rejected by the Academy of Sciences. Throughout his life Rousseau often earned his living by copying music. In Paris in the 1740's he entered literary society and wrote both the words and music for an opera *Les Muses galantes*. Rousseau lived for thirty years with an uneducated servant girl who bore him five children, according to his *Confessions;* all of them were given to an orphanage in infancy.

In 1749 Rousseau burst into prominence by winning an essay contest on the theme: "Has the progress of the arts and sciences contributed more to the corruption or purification of morals?" Rousseau criticized social institutions for having corrupted the essential goodness of nature and the human heart. In his "Discourse on the Origin of Inequality" he elaborated on the process of how social institutions must have developed into the extreme inequities of aristocratic France where the nobility and the church lived in luxury while the poor peasants had to pay most of the taxes, and in his "Discourse on Political Economy" he suggested remedies for these injustices. In 1756 he retreated to a simple country life and wrote a romantic novel *La Nouvelle Héloise* which won the hearts of many. Some historians consider Rousseau the initiator of the romantic rebellion in art and literature.

Rousseau's two greatest works were published in 1762 — *The Social Contract* and *Emile* or *On Education*. For Rousseau society itself is an implicit agreement to live together for the good of everyone with individual equality and freedom. However, people have enslaved themselves by giving over their power to governments which are not truly sovereign because they do not promote the general will. Rousseau believed that only the will of all the people together granted sovereignty. Various forms of government are instituted to legislate and enforce the laws. He wrote, "The first duty of the legislator is to make the laws conformable to the general will, the first rule of public economy is that the administration of justice should be conformable to the laws." His natural political philosophy echoes the way of Lao Tzu: "The greatest talent a ruler can possess is to disguise his power, in order to render it less odious, and to conduct the State so peaceably as to make it seem to have no need of conductors." Rousseau valued his citizenship in Geneva where he was born, and he was one of the first strong voices for democratic principles. "There can be no patriotism without liberty, no liberty without virtue, no virtue without citizens; create citizens, and you have everything you need; without them, you will have nothing but debased slaves, from the rulers of the State downwards." Rousseau goes on to explain that citizens depend upon education. *Emile* was a revolutionary book in regard to educational theory. Rousseau described how a boy can learn most naturally by direct experience. Rousseau recommended awakening the inner goodness that comes from the heart and warned against the evil contrivances of "civilized" society.

Where are there laws, and where are they respected?
Everywhere you have seen only individual interest
and men's passions reigning under this name.
But the eternal laws of nature and order do exist.
For the wise man, they take the place of positive law.
They are written in the depth of his heart
by conscience and reason. It is to these
that he ought to enslave himself in order to be free.
The only slave is the man who does evil,
for he always does it in spite of himself.

Freedom is found in no form of government;
it is in the heart of the free man.
He takes it with him everywhere.
The vile man takes his servitude everywhere.

Yet Rousseau was not against positive law. On the contrary, laws protect those who are free from the vile enslaved man who violates them. We are free within the law, but again the laws must be in harmony with reason and the general good.

Rousseau's political writings stirred up controversy, and threatened by the established powers he fled into exile to Prussia and also visited David Hume in England. Later he was able to return to France. In 1768 a populist revolt protested for more rights against an oligarchy of twenty-five councillors in Geneva. Rousseau counseled against violence but encouraged them in their struggle and predicted, "I foresee that in ten or twenty years the times will be far more favorable to the cause of the Representative party." In fact the American Revolution was about ten years away and the French Revolution about twenty. Rousseau discussed many different forms of government and indicated that there are various factors to consider in deciding on the best form of government for any given State. Generally he favored "elective aristocracy" — not hereditary but republican. In his *Constitutional Project for Corsica* he advised them to adopt democratic government and to abolish hereditary nobility. Consulted on Poland's government he recommended the gradual enfranchisement of the serfs and a multi-level civil service system whereby one could advance by merit.

In pain often from a prostatic disorder Rousseau's moodiness and paranoia of other influential people increased in his later years. Fearing distortions of his life by others which actually were written later, Rousseau tried to tell all honestly in his *Confessions* and other autobiographical works. He died on July 2, 1778.

Rousseau's writing about a federation to establish lasting peace was actually a summary and critique of a plan devised by the Abbé de Saint-Pierre (1658-1743). In 1754 an admirer of the late Abbé, Madame Dupin, suggested to Rousseau that he bring to life the good ideas in Saint-Pierre's writings. In his *Confessions* Rousseau gives his reasons for taking up the project. "Not being confined to the functions of a translator, I was at liberty sometimes to think for myself; and I had it in my power to give such a form to my work, that many important truths would pass in it under the name of the Abbé de Saint-Pierre, much more safely than under mine." He also explains why he felt Saint-Pierre's ideas were not effective. "In the offices of all the ministers of state the Abbé de St. Pierre had ever been considered as a kind of preacher rather than a real politician, and he was allowed to say what he pleased, because it appeared that nobody listened to him." It is noteworthy that out of the twenty-three volumes of Saint-Pierre's works Rousseau selected "Perpetual Peace" for his first essay.

Saint-Pierre was educated at a Jesuit college and studied the classics, logic, ethics, physics, mathematics, and metaphysics. He joined a strict order of monks, but had to leave it for reasons of health. He was at court from 1692 to 1718 and studied both the theory and practice of politics; he was particularly influenced by Plato, Bodin, Machiavelli, Grotius, Pufendorf, Richelieu, Doria, and Hobbes. *Paix perpetuelle* was first published in 1712, but he spent five more years revising it and the rest of his life trying to promote it.

Saint-Pierre attempted to use the philosophical methodology of Descartes in order to gain certainty by means of intuition and deduction. Examining the various means which could prevent war among European nations he infers that a federation of states is the best solution. Whereas Hobbes showed that for the protection and benefit of individuals there must be unity in the state, Saint-Pierre went a step further in reasoning that to safeguard the peace between nations there must be a unifying federation. Although accused by Rousseau of unrealistically expecting people to be rational, Saint-Pierre did recognize that passions control the actions of most people. Therefore to overcome motives of self-interest the fear of violence must be used to enforce law and justice. Foreshadowing Rousseau's ideas he posits that society protects people from violence by a contract and can express its sovereign will by establishing a permanent federation among the states of Europe.

Rousseau begins his description of Saint-Pierre's project by expressing the feelings in his heart.

> Never did the mind of man conceive a scheme nobler, more beautiful, or more useful than that of a lasting peace between all the peoples of Europe. Never did a writer better deserve a respectful hearing than he who suggests means for putting that scheme in practice. What man, if he has a spark of goodness, but must feel his heart glow within him at so fair a prospect? Who would not prefer the illusions of a generous spirit, which overleaps all obstacles, to that dry, repulsive reason whose indifference to the welfare of mankind is ever the chief obstacle to all schemes for its attainment? . . .
> I see in my mind's eye all men joined in the bonds of love. I call before my thoughts a gentle and peaceful brotherhood, all living in unbroken harmony, all guided by the same principles, all finding their happiness in the happiness of all.

Rousseau was aware, though, of the need for hard reasoning, and he promises to prove his assertions and asks the reader not to deny what he cannot refute.

Although governments have been instituted to control private wars, Rousseau laments the national wars which are a thousand times worse. In "The Origin of Inequality" he had described how individuals joined together to avoid conflicts, but that the larger bodies reverted to even more disastrous conflicts. "Hence arose national wars, battles, murders, and reprisals, which shock nature and outrage reason; together with all those horrible prejudices which class among the virtues the honor of shedding human blood. The most distinguished men hence learned to consider cutting each other's throats a duty; at length men massacred their fellow-creatures by thousands without so much as knowing why, and committed more murders in a single day's fighting, and more violent outrages in the sack of a single town, than were committed in the state of nature during whole ages over the whole earth." To remedy these dangers a federal form of government must be devised to unite nations, as nations unite individuals, under the authority of law. In Rousseau's time this type of government was fairly new, although it did exist in the Germanic Body, the Helvetic League, and the States General (Netherlands), and the ancients had the Greek Amphictyons, the Etruscan Lucumonies, Latin *feriae,* and the city leagues of the Gauls. He points out that Europe has much in common — the history of the Roman Empire, the Christian religion, geography, blood-ties, commerce, arts, colonies, and printing. Yet the violence in practice contradicts the moral ideals and rhetoric of governments. Treaties are temporary and very unstable; there is little or no common agreements on public law; and in conflicts between nations might makes right, and weakness is taken for wrong. Nevertheless the boundaries of countries remain fairly stable due to the natural conditions of geography and culture. No one country is powerful enough ever to conquer all the others, and if nations ally together for conquest they end up fighting among themselves. The Germanic states and the Treaty of Westphalia stabilize the international situation. The conflicts which do continually agitate never seem to result in any advantage to the sovereigns. Commerce and economics tend to keep the power of states fairly balanced. Since it is so difficult for one nation to conquer others, it is easy to see that the federation would be able to force any ambitious ruler to abide by the terms of the league.

Rousseau delineates the following four necessary conditions for the success of the federation: every important power must be a member; the laws they legislate must be binding; there must be a "coercive force capable of compelling every state to obey its common resolves;" and no member may be allowed to withdraw. The plan needs five articles. The first establishes a permanent alliance with a congress, and all conflicts "shall be settled and terminated by way of arbitration or judicial pronouncement." The second article determines which nations shall have a vote, how the presidency shall pass from one to another, and how the contribution quotas shall be raised to provide for common expenses. The third declares that existing boundaries shall be permanent. The fourth specifies how violators shall be banned and forced to comply by means of the arms of all the confederates. The fifth article recommends a majority vote at the start, but three-quarters after five years, and unanimity to change the articles.

Rousseau explains how the six motives which lead to war are all removed by this plan. "These motives are: either to make conquests, or to protect themselves from aggression, or to weaken a too powerful neighbor, or to maintain their rights against attack, or to settle a difference which has defied friendly negotiation, or, lastly, to fulfill some treaty obligation." Actually the federation makes every purpose easier to accomplish except the first, that of conquest, which it most effectively deters by gathering all powers against the aggressor. Also under the alliance a country need not fear a powerful neighbor, because the alliance together has far greater power.

Sovereigns ought not to complain of losing their prerogatives, because the federation merely is forcing them to be just. Rousseau estimates that nations would save approximately half of their military budgets. He enumerates the many evils and dangers of the prevailing conditions in Europe such as injustice because of might, insecurity of nations, expenses of defense, attacks, no guarantee for international agreements, no safe or inexpensive means of obtaining justice when wronged, risk and inconvenience of wars, loss of trade during crises, and general impoverishment and lack of security. The benefits of arbitration are: certainty of settling disputes peacefully, abolition of the causes of disputes, personal security for rulers, fulfillment of agreements between rulers, freedom of trade, smaller military expenses, increase in population, agriculture, and public wealth and happiness.

Rousseau then offers a brief critique of Saint-Pierre's project. First he wonders why it has not been adopted, and suggests that it is because the princes are short-sighted in their ambition and greed for power. They are too proud to submit themselves to arbitration; their wisdom is not equal to their confidence in good fortune in the risks of war. They are too blinded by their self-interest to see the wisdom of the general good. Rousseau recounts how Henry IV had tried to use self-interest with the powers of Europe to mold together a commonwealth, but he died. Rousseau finally concludes that the only way a federation could be established would be by means of a revolution, but sensing the violence in that he considers it as much to be feared as to be desired.

Jeremy Bentham was born February 15, 1748 in London and died there in 1832. He was the son of an attorney, and by the age of 4 he was reading and beginning to study Latin. He gained a degree at Oxford in 1763, and becoming a lawyer he criticized Blackstone, an influential legal thinker. To his father's chagrin Jeremy never practiced law or traditional politics. Instead he developed his own legal philosophy, encouraged social reform, and wrote thousands of pages codifying laws. His most famous work *An Introduction to the Principles of Morals and Legislation* was circulated among his friends and finally published in 1789. A practical thinker, he founded the utilitarian philosophy which seeks "the greatest happiness of the greatest number." He defined utility as "that property in any object whereby it tends to produce pleasure, good or happiness, or to prevent the happening of mischief, pain, evil or unhappiness to the party whose interest is considered." By means of this "hedonic calculus" he attempted to measure the positive and negative consequences of any decision. He went beyond a simple hedonism by describing six characteristics of the pleasure or pain to bring a qualitative evaluation into the quantification. One must consider therefore the intensity, duration, certainty, and nearness of the pleasure or pain. In addition the results of the pleasure or pain can be estimated in terms of fecundity and purity; fecundity means whether there will be further pleasures or pains later, and purity whether pleasures or pains are likely to be followed by their opposites. Finally one must consider the extent in terms of how many people may be affected. Bentham used these principles in deciding on the appropriate punishments for various crimes. In prison reform he sought to have "morals reformed, health preserved, industry invigorated, instruction diffused." In 1792 he was made a French citizen, and he advised that new government as well as that of the United States of America. He influenced many who were called "Benthamites," particularly James Mill and his son John Stuart Mill who wrote on Utilitarianism.

Bentham's essay "A Plan for a Universal and Perpetual Peace" was published a year after his death in *The Principles of International Law,* but he wrote it in 1789. Bentham declares that the whole world is his domain and that the press is his only tool. Everyone suffers from war, and the wise consider it the chief cause of suffering. Bentham's plan has two main propositions: 1) the reduction of military forces in Europe, and 2) the emancipation of colonies. He emphasizes the importance of a peace proposal, even if the world is not ready for it, because in that case there is a great need for ideas on peace. He asks for the prayers of Christians, and for the welfare of all civilized nations he has three goals: "simplicity of government, national frugality, and peace." Bentham proposes that it is not in the interest of Great Britain or France to have colonies, alliances, or a large navy. Perpetual treaties ought to limit troops and establish a common court of judicature to decide differences. However, Bentham is clearly pacifistic in stipulating that the court not be armed with coercive powers. As he states later on, he relies upon the power of public opinion. For this reason he was especially perturbed by the secrecy of British foreign affairs, such that he had to read the *Leyden Gazette* to get any news about British diplomacy, as there was none in the home press. Therefore he argues strongly against secrecy in international relations.

The colonies cause nothing but trouble for England and France and should be given up. It is in the interest of the mother-country because of the danger of war, military expense, corruption by patronage, and complication of government. He cites Gibraltar and the East Indies specifically. It is also better for the colonies themselves to be self-governing. Neither are alliances in the interest of Great Britain, because they lead to wars; also treaties to give advantage in trade are artificial economically and are not useful in the long run. The naval forces need only be strong enough to defend commerce against pirates. The pacification treaties which are to limit the number of troops are to be publicly announced. Bentham describes the folly of attempting conquest and the madness of war. In modern times it is useless to the people. He refers to the war between France and England from 1755 to 1763. "The struggle betwixt prejudice and humanity produced in conduct a result truly ridiculous. Prejudice prescribed an attack upon the enemy in his own territory, — humanity forbade the doing him any harm. Not only nothing was gained by these expeditions, but the mischief done to the country invaded was not nearly equal to the expense of the invasion." Trade is always advantageous to both parties, but war is ruinous.

Establishing a judicial court is in the interest of all. Bentham recommends a Congress of deputies from each country which shall be public in its proceedings. Its power is in reporting its decisions to public opinion. Here Bentham appears to be excessively idealistic in comparison to Saint-Pierre and Rousseau who felt the need for enforcement. Bentham naively believes that if secrecy were given up, the public would no longer support wars. He points to the example of the Swedish soldiers who refused to fight Russia. His pacifist ideas are not wrong, but they would depend upon an enlightened public opinion. He declares that the plunging of a nation into war against its will by ministers is not only mischievous but unconstitutional. He points out that punishing the authors of war does little good for the people of the nation. Since the warmakers cannot effectively be punished, they ought to be abandoned by the people. However, Bentham considers this not possible in his time. In war individual crimes are greatly multiplied, yet they win the approval of people. Since ministers are not deterred from misconduct, they are easily seduced by ambition and greed into wars, especially when shielded by secrecy.

Bentham's plan is quite sketchy and obviously not comprehensive, but he does show the usefulness of disarmament and the dangers of colonialism. He senses the power of public opinion but also sees how effectively it was squelched in his time. He does not really present the executive and legislative powers of a federal system, as do Saint-Pierre and Rousseau, but he does establish the principles of an international judiciary and open public opinion on international affairs.

Immanuel Kant was born on April 22, 1724 at Königsberg in East Prussia and lived his whole life there. His parents were pious and emphasized inward morality. In 1740 he entered the University of Königsberg in theology, but he also studied physics. After his father died in 1746 he worked for nine years as a family tutor. He lectured at the university on physics, mathematics, logic, metaphysics, moral philosophy, geography, and natural sciences. In 1770 he was appointed to the chair of logic and metaphysics. After working on it for a decade, in 1781 he published his *magnum opus,* the *Critique of Pure Reason.* Here he analyzed how the mind itself structures our understanding of reality by conceptual categories. More books followed, and Kant is considered by many to be the greatest philosopher of the age of enlightenment. For Kant, God, freedom, and immortality are transcendental ideas essential to the moral life. In his ethical works he formulated the categorical imperative as a guide for conduct: "Act only on that maxim through which you can at the same time will that it should become a universal law." Kant never ceased to marvel at "the starry heavens above and the moral law within." His lectures were popular, and he followed a regular routine. His daily walks were so punctual that the people of Königsberg could set their watches by his regular appearance. The only time he was known to have missed his daily walk was when he became absorbed in reading Rousseau's *Emile.* He died on February 12, 1804, and his last words were: "It is good."

Kant's philosophy had a critical perspective, and he shows how by using higher human reason and justice we can transcend the brutal strife and arguments of war.

Without the control of criticism, reason is, as it were, in a state of nature, and can only establish its claims and assertions by *war.* Criticism, on the contrary, deciding all questions according to the fundamental laws of its own institution, secures to us the peace of law and order, and enables us to discuss all differences in the more tranquil manner of a legal *process.* In the former case, disputes are ended by *victory*, which both sides may claim and which is followed by a hollow armistice; in the latter, by a *sentence*, which, as it strikes at the root of all speculative differences, ensures to all concerned a lasting peace.

In *The Science of Right* Kant discusses the right of nations and international law and also the universal right of mankind. Ethically, people ought to be treated as ends in themselves and not mechanically as a means to some end. Therefore the ruler has no right to treat his people as objects for some warlike purpose. "As such they must give their free consent, through their representatives, not only to the carrying on of war generally, but to every separate declaration of war." Kant defines three rights of peace: neutrality, guarantee, and alliance. Neutrality is the right to remain at peace when a war is nearby. Guarantee is "the right to have peace secured so that it may continue when it has been concluded." Alliance is the right of federation, that states may *defend* themselves in common against attack. However, there is no right of alliance for external aggression or internal aggrandizement. Kant applies the categorical imperative to the relations of states and rejects any action or policy which "would make a state of peace among the nations impossible." Kant points out that nations, like individuals, must enter into a legal state, in this case, a union of states, which is the only way to establish peace and the public right of nations. Thus a permanent congress of nations must eventually become practical so that differences may be settled by means of a civil process instead of by barbarous war. Kant bases the right to a universal peaceful union of all nations on the juridical principle of legal justice rather than on the moral ideal of the philanthropic or ethical principles. Because all people originally share the soil of the earth, they have a right to associate with each other. Even though perpetual peace may not be real yet, Kant emphasizes that we must work to realize it, as it is our duty. He concludes, "The universal and lasting establishment of peace constitutes not merely a part, but the whole final purpose and end of the science of right as viewed within the limits of reason."

In his "Idea for a Universal History from a Cosmopolitan

Point of View" Kant states that Nature forces people to a cosmopolitan solution making a league of nations the inevitable result of social evolution. Until then man must suffer the cruelty of conflicts. The answer lies in a moral order which can only be brought about through education. This enlightenment requires a commitment of heart to the good that is clearly understood. He laments that rulers spend little money on public education, because they spend it paying for past and future wars. Kant predicted that the ever-growing war debt (which was new in his time) will eventually make war impractical economically. He foresaw that this and the value of inter-state commerce "will prepare the way for a distant international government," even though there had never been one in world history. Looking toward the goal of world citizenship he suggested that the philosophical historian ought to note how various nations and governments have contributed to this goal.

Kant felt that war is the greatest obstacle to morality and that the preparation for war is the greatest evil; therefore we must renounce war. "The morally practical reason utters within us its irrevocable veto: *There shall be no war.*" Yet without a cosmopolitan constitution and the wisdom to voluntarily submit ourselves to its constraint, war is inevitable. The obstacles of ambition, love of power, and avarice, particularly of those in authority, stand in the way. Again education must foster the building of character in accordance with moral principles. The full realization of our destiny, the kingdom of God on earth, ultimately depends on "justice and equity, the authority, not of governments, but of conscience within us."

Kant's major work on peace entitled *Perpetual Peace* was published in 1795. He states six preliminary propositions for a perpetual peace among states:

1. No treaty of peace shall be held valid in which there is tacitly reserved matter for a future war.
2. No independent states, large or small, shall come under the dominion of another state by inheritance, exchange, purchase, or donation.
3. Standing armies shall in time be totally abolished.

4. National debts shall not be contracted with a view to the external friction of states.

5. No state shall by force interfere with the constitution or government of another state.

6. No state shall, during war, permit such acts of hostility which would make mutual confidence in the subsequent peace impossible: such are the employment of assassins, poisoners, breach of capitulation, and incitement to treason in the opposing state.

The reasons for these are fairly obvious. He adds that a state has no right to wage a punitive war, because just punishment must come from a superior authority and not an equal.

In introducing the three definitive articles, Kant observes that the state of nature tends toward conflict and war; therefore peace must be actively *established* and maintained by a civil state. Civil constitutions are of three levels: the law of men, the law of nations, and the law of world citizenship.

The first definitive article states, "The civil constitution of every state should be republican." By this Kant means that the laws must be applied to everyone universally and fairly — in other words, government by law, not by favored men. Thus the principles of freedom, common legislation, and equality must pertain. He hopes that requiring the citizens' consent to declare war will prevent its devastation, because it is usually the people, not the ruler, who sacrifices and suffers. By "republican" Kant means representative of the people, but not necessarily democracy, which he considers more likely to be despotic than representative government by one (autocracy) or a few (aristocracy). In a pure democracy it is not possible to separate the execute power from the legislative function.

The second definitive article states, "The law of nations shall be founded on a federation of free states." This constitution establishes the rights of states through a league of nations. Victory in war goes to the stronger, but it does not settle what is right. At its conclusion a peace treaty ends that war, but to end all wars forever there must be a league of peace. The more republics associate with each other, the more practical a federation becomes. In the federation a supreme legislative, executive, and judiciary power may be established to reconcile the differences between nations peaceably. But if nations do not acknowledge these supreme powers, then how can they safeguard their rights? Using unilateral maxims through force leads to "perpetual peace in the vast grave that swallows both the atrocities and their perpetrators." Therefore states must give up their savage (lawless) freedom in order to find a greater freedom and security within the constraints of public law.

The third definitive article states, "The law of world citizenship shall be limited to conditions of universal hospitality." Everyone has the right not to be treated as an enemy when arriving in another land. Kant does not consider a law of world citizenship "high-flown" or "exaggerated" but rather "indispensable for the maintenance of the public human rights and hence also of perpetual peace." How prophetic he was when he wrote, "The narrower or wider-community of the peoples of the earth has developed so far that a violation of rights in one place is felt throughout the world."

The guarantee for perpetual peace, for Kant, is the design and process of world history which we call "providence." People have spread throughout the earth and have been forced to develop lawful relations with each other. States were formed for defense against violations, and man has been forced to be good for the sake of others by laws to keep the peace. Although differences of language and religion have kept states separate, competition nevertheless maintains an equilibrium, and commerce has made peace far preferable to war.

Kant argues that politics must eventually be moral, because the moral laws are eternal and transcendent of political strategems. Like Bentham, Kant emphasizes that justice must be public and open to scrutiny. He reasons that political maxims must be able to be public in order to be legitimate; and those which are in need of publicity in order to succeed are both right and politically advantageous, because they must be in accord with the public's universal good. Therefore it is our duty to publically promote those policies which lead to the universal good of lasting peace.

81

11

Emerson's Transcendentalism and Thoreau's Civil Disobedience

"Love is the adamantean shield which makes blows ridiculous."
Ralph Waldo Emerson

"The manhood that has been in war
must be transferred to the cause of peace,
before war can lose its charm,
and peace be venerable to men."
Ralph Waldo Emerson

"Whenever we see the doctrine of peace embraced by a nation,
we may be assured it will not be one that invites injury;
but one, on the contrary, which has a friend
in the bottom of the heart of every man,
even of the violent and the base;
one against which no weapon can prosper;
one which is looked upon as the asylum of the human race
and has the tears and the blessings of mankind."
Ralph Waldo Emerson

"Only the defeated and deserters go to the wars,
cowards that run away and enlist."
Henry David Thoreau

"Men make an arbitrary code, and because it is not right,
they try to make it prevail by might.
The moral law does not want any champion.
Its asserters do not go to war.
It was never infringed with impunity."
Henry David Thoreau

"The law will never make men free;
it is men who have got to make the law free.
They are the lovers of law and order,
who observe the law when the government breaks it."
Henry David Thoreau

*"If a thousand men were not to pay their tax-bills this year,
that would not be a violent and bloody measure,
as it would be to pay them, and enable the State
to commit violence and shed innocent blood.
This is, in fact, the definition of a peaceable revolution,
if any such is possible."*

Henry David Thoreau

A forerunner of the Transcendentalists who preached against war was the Unitarian William Ellery Channing (1780-1842). Channing, like Emerson, disliked sectarian squabbles, and he was praised by Emerson above all other ministers. Channing preached in Boston from 1803 to the end of his life, and he was active in the peace movement which began in 1815 when Noah Worcester founded the Massachusetts Peace Society, the first influential peace society in the world.

In his *Discourses on War* Channing describes the miseries and crimes of war, their causes and some possible remedies. In addition to the suffering and destruction he points out how war corrupts the morals of society, promotes "criminal modes of subsistence," and endows government with dangerous powers. The sources of war are the human propensity for excitement, the lust for power, admiration for warlike deeds, false patriotism, and the upbringing and education which glamorizes military exploits. Channing sees the remedies as well as the causes to be of a moral nature. We must honor rulers and nations for their justice, benevolence, and educational institutions, not for their foreign conquests. We must learn to admire the heroes of conscience, human rights, the martyrs for peace and freedom, more than the false attributes of military courage. The peaceful qualities of the Christian teachings ought to be emphasized. Channing always stressed the inward morality. "No calculations of interest, no schemes of policy can do the work of love, of the spirit of human brotherhood. There can be no peace without but through peace within."

Channing did not follow the teaching of Jesus regarding not resisting one who is evil; he took a common-sense approach and felt that war could be justifiable by necessity. However, each citizen must inquire into the justice of the cause for which he is to fight, and he is "bound to withhold his hand if his conscience condemns the cause." Like the Transcendentalists, Channing urged self-reliance. "There is no moral worth in being swept away by a crowd, even towards the best objects." Channing warned that the attitude of rulers and nations towards foreign states which is usually partial and unjust ought to show us that war is rarely just or necessary. Channing advises the Christian to refuse war and to submit if necessary to prison and execution in martyrdom for peace. We must distinguish between reasonable laws and those which require a person "to commit manifest crimes." Every individual is responsible for his own actions, even if the rulers claim the "right of war." In a republican government the rights of speech, press, and peaceful methods of redressing public grievances are extremely valuable. Even in war these freedoms are of great importance. Channing tempers the right of free discussion with the admonition to speak and write only the truth. His sermons and writings were a strong voice for peace on earth.

Ralph Waldo Emerson was born on May 25, 1803 in Boston, Massachusetts; he was the son of a Unitarian minister. He graduated from Harvard College in 1821. Emerson married in 1829, but his wife died less than a year and a half later. At this point he doubted his beliefs and profession as a minister, and he decided to resign, stating that it was because of the eucharist. In 1832 he went to Europe where he met such noteworthies as Wordsworth, Coleridge, and Carlyle. Emerson gave public lectures, and in 1836 he published *Nature.* He had become the sage of Concord, and the literary colleagues gathering around him became known as the Transcendental Club. Emerson's inspiring lectures, essays, and poems elucidated a philosophy of life based on the inner resources of the self and revelation from the divine presence of the soul. "Trust yourself," he would say, and live spontaneously and freely in harmony with nature. He described the spiritual laws of life in essays like "Compensation," "Spiritual Laws," "Love," "Self-Reliance," and "The Over-Soul." He found his own insights echoed in the Hindu scriptures and the Romantic poets. He urged an American renaissance of culture and influenced writers such as Thoreau, Whitman, Hawthorne, and the Alcott family. He believed that culture was a way of modulating violence. Violence is not power, but the absence of power. He concluded "Self-Reliance" with these words: "Nothing can bring you peace but yourself. Nothing can bring you peace but the triumph of principles."

At the age of twelve Emerson produced the following couplet on the Revolutionary War:

Fair Peace triumphant blooms on golden wings,
And War no more of all his victories sings.

In 1832 he heard the "very good views" of Channing at a peace meeting. Emerson critized the Mexican War which he felt was caused chiefly by the interests of the slave states, and he prophesied that there would be retribution for the nation just as there is for any private felon. In a discussion with Thomas Carlyle at Stonehenge a few years later, Emerson put forward the pacifist philosophy of non-resistance and non-cooperation with governments which institutionalize violence, as an indigenous American conviction; this idea was championed by the abolitionist William Lloyd Garrison and others who would not compromise on this point as Channing had. Emerson gave one or two anecdotes which made an impression on Carlyle, and concluded, "T'is certain as God liveth, the gun that does not need another gun, the law of love and justice alone, can effect a clean revolution."

For Emerson, the soul transcends all conflict and has no enemies; soldiers he considered to be ridiculous. War is "abhorrent to all right reason" and against human progress. From the perspective of spiritual oneness he spoke of "the blazing truth that he who kills his brother commits suicide." He looked at the Civil War as a retribution to purge the nation of the evil of slavery; he detested the lack of freedom during the war, and in 1865 he vowed that if martial law came to Concord he would disobey it or move elsewhere. He foresaw "that dream of good men not yet come to pass, an International Congress." Prophetic also was this: "As if the earth, water, gases, lightning and caloric had not a million energies, the discovery of any one of which could change the art of war again, and put an end to war by the exterminating forces man can apply."

In 1838 Emerson delivered an address to the Boston meeting of the American Peace Society which has been published under the title "War" and contains his thinking on the issues of war and peace. He describes war as "an epidemic insanity, breaking out here and there like the cholera or influenza, infecting men's brains instead of their bowels." He could see that violence was dangerously contagious. War, for Emerson, is part of wild and primitive societies, and the primitive stages of religion lead to religious wars. "It is the ignorant and childish part of mankind that is the fighting part." Cruelty and violence are juvenile, and the mature spirit renounces them. Like others, Emerson notes that trade works against war, because it gives people contact, knowledge, and familiarity with their enemies. The development of learning, art, and religion make war seem like fratricide, and he adds that it is. History depicts the slow mitigation and decline of war. Yet the doctrine of the right of war still remains.

Emerson asks the perennial question — Cannot we have love instead of hate, peace instead of war? This idea, he points out, was not invented by St. Pierre nor Rousseau, but it is "the rising of the general tide in the human soul — and rising highest, and first made visible, in the most simple and pure souls, who have therefore announced it to us beforehand; but presently we all see it." Societies have been formed on this thought, and the hopes and prayers for peace are preparing for its actualization. Though it appears to be visionary to most, the idea is growing in influence and is inevitable. "War is on its last legs; and a universe peace is as sure as is the prevalence of civilization over barbarism, of liberal governments over feudal forms. The question for us is only *How soon?*" What is good and true will eventually prevail. The wise learn to trust ideas over circumstances, for appearances depend on the mind. "Every nation and every man instantly surround themselves with a material apparatus which exactly corresponds to their moral state, or their state of thought." Our war-establishments "serve as an index to show where man is now; what a bad, ungoverned temper he has; what an ugly neighbor he is; how his affections halt; how low his hope lies." However, friendly attitudes can change all this and make weapons things of the past to be displayed only in museums. Emerson delineates three stages of cultivation in regard to war and peace.

> At a certain stage of his progress, the man fights, if he be of a sound body and mind. At a certain higher stage, he makes no offensive demonstration, but is alert to repel injury, and of an unconquerable heart. At a still higher stage, he comes into the region of holiness; passion has passed away from him; his warlike nature is all converted into an active medicinal principle; he sacrifices himself, and accepts with alacrity wearisome tasks of denial and charity; but, being attacked, he bears it and turns the other cheek, as one engaged, throughout his being, no longer to the service of an individual but to the common soul of all men.

Emerson answers the common criticism of non-resistance even to the extent of not defending oneself or one's family against robbers and assassins. This, he says, only looks at the passive side of the friend of peace. Lovers of peace obviously do not choose to be plundered or slain, and if they accept martyrdom it is for

> some active purpose, some equal motive, some flaming love. If you have a nation of men who have risen to that height of moral cultivation that they will not declare war or carry arms, for they have not so much madness left in their brains, you have a nation of lovers, of benefactors, of true, great and able men. Let me know more of that nation; I shall not find them defenseless, with idle hands swinging at their sides. I shall find them men of love, honor and truth; men of an immense industry; men whose influence is felt to the end of the earth; men whose very look and voice carry the sentence of honor and shame; and all forces yield to their energy and persuasion.

A peaceful nation is protected by its spiritual power, because everyone is its friend. In individual cases it is extremely rare that a person of peace ever attracts violence. Yet Emerson adds that the wise do not decide in advance how to respond, but follow the guidance of Nature and God.

Emerson observes that organizing societies, passing resolutions, and publishing manifestoes are not too effective, especially when the participants do not practice what they preach when put to the test. He prefers private conviction to public opinion; our hope is "increased insight" which is "accomplished by the spontaneous teaching, of the cultivated soul, in its secret experience and meditation." Thus man can expel his devils, transmute his bestial nature, hear the voice of God, and go forward in his right mind. Nor is fear the right motive for peace; nothing great can be attained by cowards. Courage must be transferred from war to the cause of peace. Individuals are responsible for themselves and should not ask for protection from the state. The man of principle cannot be coerced into any wrongdoing and will not compromise his freedom and integrity. The cause of peace is not for the cowardly preservation of the safety of the luxurious and the timid. Peace must be maintained by true heroes who are willing to stake their lives for their principle and who go beyond the traditional hero in that they will not threaten another man's life — "men who have, by their intellectual insight or else by their moral elevation, attained such a perception of their own intrinsic worth that they do not think property or their own body a sufficient good to be saved by such dereliction of principle as treating a man like a sheep." Emerson places his faith in "the search of the sublime laws of morals and the sources of hope and trust, in man, and not in books, in the present, and not in the past," and hopes that these will bring war to an end. The way this happens is of little importance, although he predicts that society and events point toward a Congress of Nations. Once the mind accepts the reign of principles the modes of expression are easily found.

Henry David Thoreau was born in Concord, Massachusetts on July 12, 1817 and died there peacefully on May 6, 1862. He was educated at Harvard (1833-37) where he developed his love for Greek and Roman poetry, Oriental philosophy, and botany. He earned his living doing odd jobs, teaching school, and making lead pencils. He spent little time working at these though; having few wants, he made free time his greatest wealth. He loved nature, and his constant preoccupation was exploring the woods and ponds making detailed observations of plants and creatures. Emerson was his close friend, and he lived in Emerson's house for a time. Henry led a singular life, never marrying, and marching to his own drummer, as he put it. From 1845 to 1847 he lived alone in a small cabin he built by Walden Pond near Concord. He described this unique experiment in natural living in his great book *Walden,* criticizing those who "lead lives of quiet desperation" with all the superfluities of customary society. Thoreau lectured occasionally and struggled to get his writings published. His personal independence and straightforward manner was abrasive to some people, and he gained very little recognition during his lifetime. He lectured and wrote against slavery, particularly when the Fugitive Slave Law was passed in 1850 compelling northern law enforcement officials to capture and return runaway slaves. Thoreau was known to have helped some runaways, and he thought it absurd for a court to try to decide whether a man ought to be free. He defended the radical abolitionist John Brown.

By his personal example Thoreau put into practice the Transcendentalist principles of self-reliance, personal integrity, and spontaneous intuition. About the uplifting spiritual energy within he wrote, "I know of no more encouraging fact than the unquestionable ability of man to elevate his life by a conscious endeavor." For Thoreau philosophy was not clever logic or formulating a doctrine, "but so to love wisdom as to live according to its dictates, a life of simplicity, independence, magnamimity, and trust." He exhorted, "Explore thyself." We must learn to obey the laws of our own being which will never be in opposition to a just government. Thoreau's great innovation is in the ways he suggested for opposing an unjust government in order to be true to the higher laws of one's own being.

One day in late July of 1846 while he was living at Walden he walked into Concord to get his shoe repaired. He was met by his friend Sam Staples who was the local tax collector, constable, and jailer. Thoreau had not paid his tax for several years. Staples offerd to pay Henry's tax for him or get it reduced, but Thoreau declared that he didn't intend to pay it as a matter of principle. When Staples asked what he should do about it, Thoreau suggested that he resign his office. However, Staples replied, "Henry, if you don't pay, I shall have to lock you up pretty soon." Thoreau answered him, "As well now as any time, Sam." So Staples took him to jail. The tax was paid by someone, probably Thoreau's Aunt Maria, and Henry was released the next morning. According to Staples, Thoreau was "as mad as the devil" and did not want to leave jail, but Staples made him. He wanted to stay so he could call attention to the abolitionist cause and the Mexican War. People in Concord wanted to know the reasons for his going to jail, so Thoreau wrote out an explanation and gave it as a lecture twice in 1848. It was published in 1849 as "Resistance to Civil Government" and posthumously in 1866 as "Civil Disobedience."

Thoreau begins his essay with the well-known motto — "That government is best which governs least." This carried to its natural conclusion is no government at all, which he says will happen when people are prepared. He objects particularly to a standing army and the current "Mexican war, the work of comparatively a few individuals using the standing government as their tool." Yet Thoreau realizes that the immediate need is not for no government but for better government. "Let every man make known what kind of government would command his respect, and that will be one step toward obtaining it." Majorities usually rule because they are the strongest physically, and their policies are based upon expediency. Thoreau asks whether it is not better to decide right and wrong by conscience which everyone has. "It is not desirable to cultivate a respect for the law, so much as for the right. The only obligation which I have a right to assume, is to do at any time what I think right." But a corporation has no conscience, although conscientious people may be a corporation *with* a conscience. Undue respect for law leads to soldiers marching to the wars against their wills, common sense, and consciences. Such men have let themselves become machines, serving the state with their bodies. Others, like lawyers and politicians, serve the state with their heads. A few, reformers and martyrs, serve the state with their consciences also, but they are usually treated as enemies.

Thoreau declares that he cannot associate with the American

government, because it is a slave's government. He appeals to the right of revolution and the case of 1775. He laments, "A sixth of the population of a nation which has undertaken to be the refuge of liberty are slaves." It has become a military state, and honest men ought to rebel. He criticizes not only southern slave-owners but northern merchants and farmers who care more about commerce and agriculture than they do about humanity. Thousands are against slavery and the war, but they do nothing about it. Voting, he says, is like playing a game with right and wrong. Voting for the right does nothing for it if the majority passes the expedient instead. Thoreau accurately predicts that by the time the majority abolishes slavery there will be no slavery left to abolish. Although it is not necessarily a man's duty to work to eradicate a wrong, it is his duty not to support practically a wrong. We must not only refuse to fight in an unjust war, but also refuse to support the unjust government which conducts the war. Thoreau suggests that individuals refuse to pay their quota into the treasury.

"Action from principle, the perception and the performance of right, changes things and relations; it is essentially revolutionary." When unjust laws exist, there are three choices: 1) obey them, 2) obey them while working to change them, 3) transgress them at once. Yet the evil resulting from breaking an unjust law is the fault of the government. Thoreau wonders why government resists reform. "Why does it always crucify Christ, and excommunicate Copernicus and Luther, and pronounce Washington and Franklin rebels?" Thoreau advises us to let minor injustices pass if the remedy is worse than the evil; "but if it is of such a nature that it requires you to be the agent of injustice to another, then, I say, break the law. Let your life be a counter friction to stop the machine. What I have to do is to see, at any rate, that I do not lend myself to the wrong which I condemn." If a person is truly in the right, he has God on his side and constitutes a majority of one. His contact with the tax collector was Thoreau's only association with the government and therefore his best means of protest. The action of one honest man can do more for reform than all the words in the world. "Under a government which imprisons any unjustly, the true place for a just man is also a prison." The person who has experienced a little injustice for the sake of justice is more effective, as truth is stronger than error. Thoreau exhorts us:

> Cast your whole vote, not a strip of paper merely, but your whole influence. A minority is powerless while it conforms to the majority; it is not even a minority then; but it is irresistible when it clogs by its whole weight. If the alternative is to keep all just men in prison, or give up war and slavery, the State will not hesitate which to choose.

Thoreau treats of imprisonment instead of the seizure of property, because he believes that people of principle are usually poor, while the rich have sold themselves to the institution; they enjoy Caesar's government and neglect God. It is not necessary to rely on the protection of the state. When the state is corrupt it is no shame to be poor, and disobedience is more worthy than obeying.

In prison Thoreau thought of the absurdity of confining his body when his mind and spirit are free, and he pitied the state for trying to punish his body because they could not get at him. They use superior physical strength against his body, but moral force comes from a higher law. When a government şays, "Your money or your life," it is playing the thief. Why should one give in to that? Thoreau describes his stay in prison and the changed attitude of the townspeople to him when he came out. He also mentioned that he never refused to pay the highway tax or support the schools, but he must refuse allegiance to the State. Those whose taxes support the State at war are helping injustice. Thoreau expresses an eagerness to conform to the laws of the land so long as there is no moral principle to be violated. He is willing to obey those who know more than he; yet the authority of the government depends upon the consent of the governed. "There will never be a really free and enlightened State, until the State comes to recognize the individual as a higher and independent power, from which all its own power and authority are derived, and treats him accordingly."

Thoreau's essay had little impact in the nineteenth century, but in the twentieth it has become a manual for social protest. Leo

Tolstoy noticed it and asked Americans why they did not pay more attention to Thoreau's ideas instead of their financial and industrial millionaries and their generals and admirals. Mahatma Gandhi put civil disobedience into practice on a mass scale in South Africa and India; Martin Luther King, Jr. used the techniques in the civil rights movement, and anti-war activists have also applied these principles, as we shall see in later chapters.

12
Religion for World Peace: Bahá'u'lláh and 'Abdu'l-Bahá

*"These strifes and this bloodshed and discord must cease,
and all men be as one kindred and one family."*

Bahá'u'lláh

*"It is not for him to pride himself
who loveth his own country,
but rather for him who loveth the whole world.
The earth is but one country, and mankind its citizens."*

Bahá'u'lláh

*"The Great Being, wishing to reveal the prerequisites
of the peace and tranquility of the world
and the advancement of its peoples, hath written:
The time must come when the imperative necessity
for the holding of a vast, an all-embracing assemblage of men
will be universally recognized.
The rulers and kings of the earth must needs attend it,
and, participating in its deliberations,
must consider ways and means as will lay
the foundations of the world's Great Peace amongst men.
Such a peace demandeth that the Great Powers should resolve,
for the sake of the tranquility of the peoples of the earth,
to be fully reconciled among themselves.
Should any king take up arms against another,
all should unitedly arise and prevent him."*

Bahá'u'lláh

*"There is not one soul whose conscience does not testify
that in this day there is no more important matter
in the world than that of Universal Peace."*

'Abdu'l-Bahá

*"I charge you all that each one of you concentrate
all the thoughts of his heart on love and unity.
When a thought of war comes,
oppose it by a stronger thought of peace.
A thought of hatred must be destroyed*

by a more powerful thought of love.
When soldiers of the world draw their swords to kill,
soldiers of God clasp each other's hands.
So may all the savagery of men disappear
by the mercy of God, working through
the pure in heart and the sincere of soul."

'Abdu'l-Bahá

The Bahá-í faith began in Persia in the middle of the nineteenth century. On May 23, 1844 Mírzá 'Alí Muhammad declared that he was the **Báb (Gate)** — "the channel of grace from some great Person still behind the veil of glory." He was a forerunner as John the Baptist had been for the Christ. Gathering eighteen disciples he went on pilgrimage to Mecca where his oratory and inspired writings encouraged his followers and alarmed the orthodox Muslim authorities. They persuaded the Governor of Fars to persecute the heretics, and the **Báb** was subjected to imprisonments, deportations, examinations before tribunals, torture, and finally a firing squad in 1850. After the first round of shots, the **Báb** and his companion were unhurt; the bullets had merely cut the ropes by which they were suspended. The **Báb** talked for a while with his friends in a nearby room, while the Armenians who made up the firing squad refused to fire again because they believed he was saved by a miracle. However, another regiment of soldiers was ordered to fire, and his martyrdom was completed. This event stimulated even more people to follow his teachings, but the persecutions continued with more than 20,000 people losing their lives.

Mirzá Husayn 'Alí who became known as **Bahá'u'lláh** (Glory of God) was born about two years before the **Báb** on November 12, 1817 in Teheran. Although given no formal education he impressed everyone with his wisdom and knowledge. When he was twenty-two and his father died, it was expected that he would take up his father's prestigious position in the government, but the young man had other ideas. His son, who was to become known as 'Abdu-l-Bahá (Servant of Bahá), was born on the same day as the Báb's declaration. **Bahá'u'lláh** became one of the leading Bábís and was imprisoned and tortured for the cause. He was exiled to Baghdad and spent two years alone in the wilderness. When he returned to the city of Baghdad, his teachings attracted not only Muslims but also Jews, Christians, and Zoroastrians. Because of his popularity, in 1863 the Persian government requested the Turkish government to order him to Constantinople. His followers were upset, and while camping in a garden outside the city for twelve days in preparation for the journey, Bahá'u'lláh announced that he was the Promised One foretold by the Báb. A majority of the Bábís who accepted his mission became known as Bahá'ís. He was moved from Constantinople to Adrianople; from there he sent his famous proclamations to the current world leaders including Napoleon III, Czar Alexander II, Queen Victoria, Kaiser Wilhelm I, Emperor Francis Joseph, Sultán 'Abdu'l-Azíz, Násiri'd-Dín Sháh, the rulers of America, the elected representatives of the people, Pope Pius IX, and the clergy and people of various faiths. In these exhortations he pleaded for peace and the unity of mankind.

O Rulers of the earth! Be reconciled among yourselves, that ye may need no more armaments save in a measure to safeguard your territories and dominions. Beware lest ye disregard the counsel of the All-Knowing, the Faithful.

Be united, O Kings of the earth, for thereby will the tempest of discord be stilled amongst you, and your people find rest, if ye be of them that comprehend. Should any one among you take up arms against another, rise ye all against him, for this is naught but manifest justice.

In 1868 Bahá'u'lláh was sent to 'Akká (Acre) in Palestine where he spent the rest of his life under arrest, though he eventually was allowed to reside in a mansion which had been abandoned during a plague. He died on May 29, 1892, and in his will declared that his son, 'Abdu'l-Bahá was to be his representative and expounder of his teachings.

Bahá'u'lláh continually taught that true religion recognizes the unity of mankind and promotes the love of all humanity. Prejudices based on religion, race, or nationality are contrary to spirituality and divine love. He prophesied that civilization is moving toward world unity. The earth is one, and the servant of God is dedicated to the service of the entire human race. Even though his followers were persecuted, he advised peaceful non-resistance toward violence. Reconstructing the world does not require the use of weapons but rather a firm adherence to justice and faith in God. "Such hath been the patience, the calm, the resignation and contentment of this people that they have become the exponents of justice, and so great hath been their forbearance, that they have suffered themselves to be killed rather than kill." Bahá'u'lláh explains that they can do this because of their trust in God. Nevertheless to attain world unity and peace individual nations must not be allowed to make war on others. Therefore Bahá'u'lláh recommended a world assembly so that all the nations together could prevent aggression. He believed that this is divinely ordained and that in time people would come to recognize it. All the leaders of the earth must participate and join together to maintain with their collective power peace and justice. Bahá'u'lláh described the political unity of states as the Lesser Peace while the Most Great Peace requires spiritual unity in addition to political and economic cooperation. Bahá'u'lláh outlined a plan with a House of Justice to make lawful decisions. He suggested the use of a universal language and education for everyone.

The teachings of Bahá'u'lláh were expressed in more detail by his son 'Abdu'l-Bahá, particularly when he traveled to Europe and America from 1911 to 1913. 'Abdu'l-Bahá also exhorted everyone to realize the unity of mankind and practice love and spiritual brotherhood. "The time has come when all mankind shall be united, when all races shall be loyal to one fatherland, all religions become one religion and racial and religious bias pass away. It is a day in which the oneness of humankind shall uplift its standard and international peace like the true morning flood the world with its light." For 'Abdu'l-Bahá any religion which causes hatred and division is no religion at all and to withdraw from such a religion is a religious act. Likewise race prejudice is an illusion created by man, because God created one human race and He wishes all colors to share His blessings. We must practice the divine religion of love and unity or else restrictive dogmas and bigotry will lead to strife and warfare, threatening the destruction of the human race. Love and accord dissolve dissensions and unite all in one happy family of peace and unity. Religion can be a powerful influence for peace, because it recognizes that there is one reality.

'Abdu'l-Bahá contrasts peace and war. Peace is light, life, guidance, Godly, humane, constructive, love, harmony, health, and brotherhood, while war is darkness, death, error, satanic, savage, destructive, hatred, discord, disease, and strife. Men do not need to kill other men to survive. Therefore the causes of war are to be found in greed, hatred, and selfishness. Ignorant soldiers fight for the greed and ambition of their leaders.

'Abdu'l-Bahá recounts how Bahá'u'lláh declared the Most Great Peace and the principle of international arbitration and disarmament, even though he and his followers had to suffer persecution for his criticism of leaders' selfish aims. 'Abdu'l-Bahá gives the details of his father's teachings on Universal Peace. First, the independent investigation of reality enables humanity to move toward greater truth. Second, humanity is one, and all human beings have the same divine Shepherd. Third, religion is to be the cause of fellowship and love, and any religion which causes estrangement is unnecessary. Fourth, religion must be in harmony with science and reason so that it may influence people. Fifth, "religious, racial, political, economic and patriotic prejudices destroy the edifice of humanity." Patriotic prejudices forget that the land belongs to all people and is to be shared. Sixth, a universal language may be spread to all people in order to eliminate misunderstandings. 'Abdu'l-Bahá personally commended efforts to promote the use of Esperanto. Seventh is the equality of women and men. Women must have equal opportunity to advance in science, literature, and in civil and political life. In fact, the imbalance of masculine qualities over the feminine has prevented a harmonious and peaceful society. 'Abdu'l-Bahá explained:

> The world in the past has been ruled by force, and man has dominated over woman by reason of his more forceful and aggressive qualities both of body and mind. But the

balance is already shifting; force is losing its dominance, and mental alertness, intuition, and the spiritual qualities of love and service, in which woman is strong, are gaining ascendancy. Hence the new age will be an age less masculine and more permeated with the feminine ideals, or, to speak more exactly, will be an age in which the masculine and feminine elements of civilization will be more evenly balanced.

Society is like a bird with two wings, woman and man; both wings must be equally developed for the bird to fly successfully. Eighth, the voluntary sharing of property by the wealthy eliminates conflict between the rich and poor. Ninth is human freedom — not only political but liberation from the captivity of animal drives. Tenth, religion is a tremendous power for moral education. Eleventh, the successes of material civilization must be vivified by spiritual values, as the body by the soul. Twelfth, universal education must be provided by the community, if not privately, for every child. Finally the principle of justice must be practiced, and for this Bahá'u'lláh suggested a Supreme Tribunal made up of representatives elected from every nation in proportion to population. This union of nations will decide all disputes by international arbitration. The power of the union must be used to prevent aggression by any nation. "By a general agreement all the governments of the world must disarm simultaneously." In 1914 'Abdu'l-Bahá was describing what unfortunately is still true. "As long as one nation increases her military and naval budget other nations will be forced into this crazy competition through their natural and supposed interests." It is the duty of nations to check aggressors rather than remaining neutral; world unity requires that every other nation unite against any aggressor.

'Abdu'l-Bahá looked toward the unification of the East and West, the spiritual and the material, so that there may be a paradise on earth. Peace, love, and friendship enable both science and the knowledge of God to flourish. World peace is not an impossible ideal, for everything is possible with divine benevolence. If we desire friendship with everyone on earth with all our hearts, then this ideal will spread until it reaches the minds of all people. 'Abdu'l-Bahá encourages us to practice universal love.

Be kind to all people, love humanity, consider all mankind as your relations and servants of the most high God. Strive day and night that animosity and contention may pass away from the hearts of men, that all religions shall become reconciled and the nations love each other, so that no racial, religious or political prejudice may remain and the world of humanity behold God as the beginning and end of all existence. God has created all and all return to God. Therefore love humanity with all your heart and soul.

13
Leo Tolstoy on the Law of Love

*"A Christian does not quarrel with any one,
does not attack any one, nor use violence against one;
on the contrary, he himself without murmuring bears violence;
but by this very relation to violence he not only frees himself,
but also the world from external power."*

Leo Tolstoy

*"War is so unjust and ugly that all who wage it
must try to stifle the voice of conscience within themselves."*

Leo Tolstoy

*"The evil committed by man not only weakens his soul
and deprives him of true happiness,
but more often than not
falls back on the one who commits it."*

Leo Tolstoy

*"Eventually institutional violence will disappear,
not as a result of external action,
but thanks only to the calls of conscience of men
who have awakened to the truth."*

Leo Tolstoy

*"Every man, in refusing to take part in military service
or to pay taxes to a government
which uses them for military purposes, is,
by this refusal, rendering a great service to God and man,
for he is thereby making use of the most efficacious means
of furthering the progressive movement of mankind
toward that better social order which it is striving after
and must eventually attain."*

Leo Tolstoy

Leo Tolstoy, the son of Count Nicholas Tolstoy, was born on August 28, 1828 (September 9, 1828 in our Gregorian calendar) at the family estate Yasnaya Polyana where he spent most of his life about 100 miles south of Moscow. His mother died before he was two years old, and when he was about nine, his father and grandmother died. Leo was raised by aunts and tutors, and he followed his older brothers to the University of Kazan; wanting to become a diplomat he studied in the Department of Oriental Languages and strove to become a sophisticated gentleman of the world. In 1847 he began to manage his estate at Yasnaya Polyana while also pursuing the social life in Moscow and St. Petersburg. In his diary he formulated rules for living which he had great difficulty following. At age 23 he followed his older brother Nicholas into the army life in the Caucasus, and he fought in the Crimean War until 1856. During this period he struggled with a penchant for gambling, "fits of lust" and "criminal sloth." He criticized the army for lacking loyalty, courage, and dignity, and complained about the corporal punishment inflicted on the soldiers and about the incompetence of the generals. He was only 24 when he wrote in his diary that because war is unjust those who are involved in it must stifle their consciences. He began writing sketches on *Childhood, Boyhood,* and *Youth,* short stories, and described the suffering of a civilized man amid the spontaneous lives of the natives in *The Cossacks.* He studied educational methods and started an experimental school for the local peasants. He formulated his progressive educational theories under the influence of Rousseau's writings and his travels in western Europe. When Leo was 34 he married Sonya who bore him thirteen children and assisted him in his literary career which in the next fifteen years produced two of the greatest novels ever written, *War and Peace* and *Anna Karenina.*

The epic *War and Peace* describes the lives of five aristocratic families during the Napoleonic Wars between Russia and France. His subtle psychological insights and realistic details create an entire world from various points of view. Tolstoy's own future views are foreshadowed by the esoteric philosophy of the Freemasons who initiate Pierre into their mysteries. He is exhorted to an active life of virtue, and although they endeavor to reform society, they renounce the use of violence. "Every violent reform deserves censure, for it quite fails to remedy evil while men remain what they are, and also because wisdom needs no violence." The answer lies in personal transformation which Pierre undergoes during the course of events. The moral evil of the war is summarized by Tolstoy in these words:

> An event took place opposed to human reason and to
> human nature. Millions of men perpetrated against one
> another such innumerable crimes, frauds, treacheries,
> thefts, forgeries, issues of false money, burglaries,
> incendiarisms, and murders as in whole centuries are not
> recorded in the annals of all the law courts of the world,
> but which those who committed them did not at the time
> regard as being crimes.

Tolstoy does not lay the blame on the leaders and "great men"
whom he believes are merely puppets of history, a history that is
shaped by the millions of choices made by the countless
individuals participating.

> Each man lives for himself, using his freedom to attain
> his personal aims, and feels with his whole being that he
> can do or abstain from doing this or that action; but as
> soon as he has done it, that action performed at a certain
> moment in time becomes irrevocable and belongs to
> history, in which it has not a free but a predestined
> significance.

Thus, although man lives consciously for himself, the social
unconscious of collective humanity exerts a greater influence
depending on how high the man stands on the social ladder which
in turn determines his power over others. This diagnosis was to
lead to Tolstoy's twofold solution to the problem of a violent
society — that is, the social solution of dismantling the political
institutions which by their nature force their power on the people,
and the individual solution of refusing to participate in
institutions of violence from a sense of inner conscience. In *Anna
Karenina* the Tolstoyan hero Levin declares, "The good of
society is dependent upon scrupulous obedience of the moral law
engraved in every human heart," and he also believes that "no
one, therefore, should desire or advocate war, whatever generous
aim it purports to serve."

In his *Confession* Tolstoy describes the spiritual crisis he had in
1879 when he contemplated suicide. He explains how literary

minds fall away from traditional religion only to get lost in an aesthetic nihilism. Neither science nor theology satisfied his quest for meaning in life, but living a simple and good life to benefit others awakened in him a feeling of faith in God that reasoning could not find. He returned to religion, but after a while he left the dogma and ritual of the church behind to explore for himself the original teachings of Christ especially as presented in the Sermon on the Mount. He made his own translation, harmony, and summary of the gospels and expounded their precepts in his writings for the rest of his life. He was particularly moved by the command not to resist him that is evil but to love your enemies. With this foundation he criticized the hypocrisy of Christian societies which practiced violence in warfare and criminal executions. He felt that the three causes of war in his time were the unequal distribution of property, the military establishment, and false and deceptive religion. In *What I Believe* he contrasted the teachings of Jesus to the dogma and practices of the Orthodox Church. In *What Shall We Do Then?* Tolstoy presented his observations of the slums in Moscow and analyzed the causes of poverty, In deciding what to do he suggests three things: 1) not to lie to oneself or be afraid of the truth, 2) to renounce one's sense of righteousness, prerogatives, and privileges, and 3) to labor with one's whole being to support oneself and others.

In 1891 a severe famine occurred in Russia, and visiting a friend in Ryazan Province, Tolstoy was moved to work in relief efforts, although his pleas for help were attacked by government officials. In 1897 he published *What is Art?* propounding that in good art the soul of the artist infects his audience by means of sympathetic feelings, and he hailed religious art which flows from the love of God and man as the highest art. True art encourages peaceful co-existence of people not by the external means of courts, police, and institutions, but "through the free and joyous activity of men. Art should remove violence." Art can teach people how to feel for other people and recognize the universal brotherhood of humanity so that the kingdom of love may be established.

Near the close of the century about 12,000 Dukhobors were

being persecuted in Russia because they refused to serve in the army since it is against Christian teachings. The persecutions had depleted their resources so that they did not have the funds to migrate to America. Tolstoy rapidly completed his novel *Resurrection* and turned the considerable sum of money he received from it over to the Dukhobors and along with other donations, particularly from English and American Quakers, they were able to move to Canada.

Tolstoy had adopted a new life-style after his conversion, giving all his property to his wife and living almost like a peasant. He gave up smoking and drinking and became a vegetarian. He worked in the fields, cleaned his own room and made his own boots. Because of his radical ideas he was excommunicated by the church. Finally after conflicts between his wife and the leading Tolstoyan disciple Chertkov the old man left his home at the age of 82 and died shortly after starting on this pilgrimage as a religious hermit.

Tolstoy's major book on nonviolence and the way to peace is *The Kingdom of God is Within You* which was completed in 1893. He begins by surveying the non-resistants in America such as the Quakers, William Lloyd Garrison, and Adin Ballou who dedicated their lives to these principles. He recounts how some people in Russia refused to do military service because of religious convictions. Tolstoy explains how not resisting evil with evil is the way to eliminate evil altogether.

> It alone makes it possible to tear the evil out by the root, both out of one's own heart and out of the neighbor's heart. This doctrine forbids doing that by which evil is perpetuated and multiplied. He who attacks another and insults him, engenders in another the sentiment of hatred, the root of all evil. To offend another, because he offended us, for the specious reason of removing an evil, means to repeat an evil deed, both against him and against ourselves.

Tolstoy responds to five typical criticisms of non-resistance. First, some assert that violence does not contradict Christ's teachings, believing that government is not bound by the admonitions toward humility, forgiveness, and love of enemies;

they simply quote Biblical passages to their liking and ignore the essence of the teachings. Second, people feel that turning the other cheek and giving up one's shirt is too high a moral demand for this world, and that if force were not used to stop evildoers they would destroy all the good people; however, this argument destroys the Christian teachings because true Christians do not wish to judge evil-doers, nor do they consider themselves capable of judging accurately, nor would they be willing to execute punishment. The third argument is that although one ought not to defend oneself he ought to defend his neighbors; this still contradicts Christ's teaching because Jesus did not allow his disciples to defend him and because the violence used to defend against threatened violence may be even worse since we never know what will result beforehand. Fourth, theologians and defenders of the church and state consider violations of non-resistance as accidental and even justifiable under certain circumstances such as wars and executions; yet they do not try to justify the breaking of other commandments such as against fornication, and one reason why people ignore non-resistance is because church preachers do not recognize it. The fifth device is merely to ignore the question and criticize non-resistants for being one-sided or extremists; these people are the hardest to reach, because they are not willing to discuss the issue and assume they are right without any logical justification whatsoever, being under a kind of "hypnotic suggestion."

Tolstoy delineates the following five ideals and commandments of Christ expressed in the Sermon on the Mount: 1) have no ill-will against anyone, but love all; don't even offend with a word; 2) complete chastity, even in thought; 3) live only in the present and don't worry about the future; don't swear and don't promise; 4) never use violence nor repay evil with evil, but suffer insult and give up possessions; and 5) love our enemies and those who hate us by treating them as ourselves. For Tolstoy these commandments are to be practiced now, and they will be followed by higher ones on the path to perfection. These teachings transcend the social conception of life which may be limited by exclusive love of one's family, tribe, nation, race, or even humanity. These and socialistic brotherhoods are based on the love of personality, but the Christian love ever expands because it is based on the love of God.

Tolstoy points out the contradiction of the military in a society which professes itself to be Christian — believing in the brotherhood of men and being prepared for hostility and murder — "of being at the same time a Christian and a gladiator." Tolstoy finds three prevalent attitudes to war. Those who consider it accidental and propose diplomatic and international solutions. Others deplore the horrors of war but believe that it is inevitable; these are the pessimistic writers who describe how terrible life is but offer no real solution. The third group has lost its conscience and justifies wars as part of natural evolution and the survival of the fittest. For Tolstoy even the first group which organizes societies and diplomatic methods to resolve conflicts is rather like trying to catch a bird by putting salt on his tail; the salt can only be used if the bird is as good as caught anyway. Thus international agreements will only be effective when men have decided to renounce the use of weapons. Therefore the critical step is to refuse to participate in or support military forces. Tolstoy compares the advantages and disadvantages for a person to submit or not to submit to military service and summarizes the advantages in these words:

> For him who has not refused, the advantages will consist in this, that, having submitted to all the humiliations and having executed all the cruelties demanded of him, he may, if he is not killed, receive red, golden, tin-foil decorations over his fool's garments, and he may at best command hundreds of thousands of just such bestialized men as himself, and be called a field-marshall, and receive a lot of money.
>
> But the advantages of him who refuses will consist in this, that he will retain his human dignity, will earn the respect of good men, and, above all else, will know without fail that he is doing God's work, and so an incontestable good to men.

How, then, does society make soldiers of its men? by intimidation, bribery, hypnotization, and segregation from civilian society. Observing the stirrings of revolutionary movements Tolstoy correctly predicts that the communists and socialists will put even the economic sphere under the control of the government. The Christian solution of nonviolence must be used if men are ever to free themselves from enslavement to violent institutions. Those who follow a merely social concept of life do not refuse to submit, and many fight and kill in the name of liberty, equality, and fraternity. However, the true Christian is liberated from social powers because he lives "the divine law of love, which is implanted in the soul of every man and is brought into consciousness by Christ." Although he may suffer external violence or physical imprisonment, the Christian is free (not a slave of sin) and therefore is not compelled by external threats. Freedom is not found in external things but in the inward liberation of choosing what is loving. Tolstoy cites cases where conscientious Christians refused to submit to military service and to swear such an oath or refused to pay taxes; he observes that they are more effective with peaceful disobedience than are the socialists, communists, and anarchists with their bombs, riots, and revolutions, for governments know how to handle external threats. Force can fight force, but love and peace have a subtle power all their own. He concludes, "The governments feel their indefensibleness and weakness, and the men of the Christian consciousness are awakening from their lethargy and are beginning to feel their strength.

Those who try to rule with violence are obviously breaking the golden rule and are morally inferior to those who prefer suffering violence to doing violence. The state tries to justify its violence with the assumption that it prevents violence, but Tolstoy holds that if the government stopped all its violence then the total amount of violence would decrease. Since it is the bad or morally inferior who do violence, the government has placed itself among the bad. Violence will never cease due to the threat of violence, but only when people become good and refrain from it altogether. Thus society improves as more and more people renounce the cruelty of violence. Violence distorts public opinion as to what is right and obscures people's recognition of the true spiritual forces of humanity. When public opinion condemns violence, then using violence in government becomes less desirable and those holding positions tend to use less violence. Inevitably people will eventually see the uselessness, silliness, and indecency of violence, and weapons will no longer be employed. The kingdom of God will come as we live by the light within us.

In the last fifteen years of his life Tolstoy wrote numerous articles and letters promoting the philosophy of nonviolence and the technique of civil disobedience. He expressed his gratitude to several American writers who especially influenced him, namely, Garrison, Parker, Emerson, Ballou, and Thoreau. He repeated the basic principle that murder is wrong and that killing one's fellow human beings in any circumstances is murder. Thus the simple truth is that war and executions are murder, even though people try to justify them. The essential solution to war is for people to realize what it really is and call it by its right name. "It should be understood that an army is an instrument of murder, that the recruiting and drilling of armies which Kings, Emperors, and Presidents carry on with so much self-assurance are preparations for murder." Therefore a Christian cannot be a soldier, that is, a murderer, and a man with any sense will not enslave himself to a master whose business is killing. The way to end war, then, is for those who recognize that it is wrong to refrain from fighting and even to cease supporting warlike governments by refusing to pay their taxes. Those who are not hypnotized into the wrongdoing must refuse; those who do follow reason, conscience, and God will always attain the best results for themselves and for the world. They say something like this:

What you tell us about the danger threatening us, and about your anxiety to guard us against it, is a fraud. All the states are assuring us that they desire peace, and yet at the same time all are arming themselves against the others. Moreover, according to that law, which you yourselves recognize, all men are brothers, and it makes no difference whether one belongs to this state or to that; therefore the idea of our being attacked by other nations, with which you try to frighten us, has no terror for us; we regard it as a matter of no importance. The essential thing, however, is that the law given to us by God and recognized even by you who are requiring us to participate in killing, distinctly forbids, not killing only, but also every kind of violence. Therefore we cannot, and will not, take part in your preparations for murder, we will give no money for the purpose, and we will not attend the meetings arranged by you with the object of perverting men's minds and consciences, and transforming them into instruments of violence, obedient to any bad man who may choose to make use of them.

Now the real struggle is between those who use violence and those who refuse to be violent. Thus Tolstoy urges both officers and soldiers to resign. He exposes the cruel punishments the army uses to turn men into less than animals, into machines, which perform deeds most repulsive to human nature. He exhorts men to obey God rather than the shameful commands of men.

We must learn to see through the perverted rationalizations that governments use to justify war. Tolstoy particularly warns against the dangerous sentiment of patriotism which he defines as "the preference for one's own country or nation above the country or nation of any one else" and finds it aptly illustrated in the German patriotic song, "Deutschland, Deutschland über Alles." This sentiment he regards as immoral because it violates the golden rule by trying to benefit oneself at the expense of others. In patriotism Tolstoy sees "a means of obtaining for the rulers their ambitions and covetous desires, and for the ruled the abdication of human dignity, reason, and conscience, and a slavish enthralment to those in power." Patriotism must inevitably yield to universal brotherhood. Tolstoy proposes that the most important changes in the life of humanity are not brought about by armies nor machines nor exhibitions nor labor unions nor revolutions nor inventions but by a change in public opinion. We need only to stop lying to ourselves and realize that "strength is not in force but in truth." Oppressive governments fear the clear expression of thought more than anything else; spiritual force is free and always accessible in the depths of human consciousness. We must learn to use the consciousness of truth by expressing what we know is right. By expressing the truth the new public opinion will become enlightened. This truth is found in our consciences and is given to us by God. Christ gave us his peace, but it is up to us to bring it into realization.

The heroes in this struggle for peace are the martyrs who have died for refusing to do violence or who have been locked up in prisons. Many were little known; yet the spiritual power of their actions can influence consciences of countless people. Tolstoy prophesies that war must disappear, and he sees many signs of its demise. "These signs are such as the helpless position of governments, which more and more increase their armaments; the multiplication of taxation and the discontent of the nations; the extreme degree of efficiency with which deadly weapons are constructed; the activity of congresses and societies of peace; but above all, the refusals of individuals to take military service." All of these indicators are much more pronounced now than they were in the last century. Just as slavery was recognized as wrong in the nineteenth century and was eventually eradicated, so too war is now being considered a useless, wicked, harmful madness which must also be eliminated. Those who are persecuted for the sake of peace and justice gradually awaken the consciences of their persecutors, not by coercive force but by love and persuasion. By renouncing violence the non-resistance principle recognizes the freedom of every individual to make his own decisions. By love and rational persuasion humanity can truly progress toward a better way of life. Tolstoy elucidates three ways we can know how to act. First, the collective wisdom of mankind advises us to act toward others as we would have them act toward us. Second, we can use our reason to see that if people acted in this way it would be best for everyone. Third, by listening to our hearts we know by intuition that the loving action leads to happiness.

Tolstoy's last book was *The Law of Love and the Law of Violence*. He begins the preface, "The only reason why I am writing this is because, knowing the one means of salvation for Christian humanity, from its physical suffering as well as from the moral corruption in which it is sunk, I, who am on the edge of the grave, cannot be silent." He could see the increasing conflicts between revolutionaries and governments, between oppressed nations and their oppressors, state against state and West against East, but few are aware of the remedies to these problems. Tolstoy observes that animalistic man is unhappy and that evil weakens the soul and usually rebounds. Force does not keep people social, and cruelty and lies must eventually be replaced by Christ's law of love. "It is this law of love and its recognition as a rule of conduct in all our relations with friends, enemies and offenders which must inevitably bring about the complete transformation of the existing order of things, not only among Christian nations, but among all the peoples of the globe." This obviously rules out violence. Although reason is often used to justify sin, the horrors of wars are much worse than the motives and justifications for them ever consider. Governments really use violence so that a minority may continue to exploit a majority by maintaining the established "order." The majority allows themselves to be exploited, because they are deceived and because they have no faith in God but are manipulated by considerations of self-interest. Tolstoy reiterates the need to refuse military service and describes the joy experienced by some of those he saw in prison. Although conditions in the world seem to be reaching a point where there seems to be no solution, the supreme law of love is still the way to salvation. Conscience has been the moving impulse behind the gradual evolution and recognition of human rights. The type of political or social system, whether to preserve a monarchy or a republic or replace it with a socialist or communist regime, if the method is violent, they cannot but fail until the supreme law of love is universally practiced, for love transcends all the social systems. We are free and happy according to how closely we follow the supreme law of life which is love; when everyone observes the law of love, union will be realized without effort. These ideas Tolstoy wanted to convey before he died, that by perfecting our love toward our fellow man we free ourselves from illusions.

At the end of his life Tolstoy corresponded with Mohandas Gandhi concerning the way of love and non-resistance. Two months before his death he wrote to Gandhi, "Socialism, communism, anarchism, the Salvation Army, the growth of crime, unemployment among the population, the growth of the insane luxury of the rich and the destitution of the poor, the terrible growth in the number of suicides — all these things are signs of this internal contradiction which ought to and must be solved — and, of course, solved in the sense of recognizing the law of love and renouncing all violence." He praised Gandhi's work in South Africa and reported about refusals to do military service in Russia. "However insignificant may be the number of your people who practice non-resistance and of our people in Russia who refuse military service, both can boldly say that God is with them. And God is more powerful than men." Thus the baton of peace and nonviolence passed to a humble Indian thousands of miles away whose use of the peace philosophy and nonviolent technique on a mass scale was to astound the world.

14
Mahatma Gandhi's Nonviolent Revolution

"Gandhi continues what the Buddha began.
In the Buddha the spirit of love set itself the task
of creating different spiritual conditions in the world;
in Gandhi it undertakes to transform all *worldly conditions."*
Albert Schweitzer

"Nonviolence is the law of our species
as violence is the law of the brute.
The spirit lies dormant in the brute,
and he knows no law but that of physical might.
The dignity of man requires obedience to a higher law —
to the strength of the spirit.
Mahatma Gandhi

"If man will only realize
that it is unmanly to obey laws that are unjust,
no man's tyranny will enslave him."
Mahatma Gandhi

"There can be no inward peace without true knowledge."
Mahatma Gandhi

"Science of war leads one to dictatorship pure and simple.
Science of nonviolence can alone lead one to pure democracy."
Mahatma Gandhi

"For self-defense, I would restore the spiritual culture.
The best and most lasting self-defense is self-purification."
Mahatma Gandhi

Mohandas Karamchand Gandhi was born on October 2, 1869 in western India. His father was a local politician, and his mother was a religious Vaishnavite. At the age of 13 Mohandas was married to a girl his own age and began an active sex life. After some undistinguished education it was decided that he should go to England to study law. He gained his mother's permission by promising to refrain from wine, women, and meat, but he defied his caste's regulations which forbade travel to England. He joined the Inner Temple law college in London. In searching for a vegetarian restaurant he discovered its philosophy in Henry Salt's *A Plea for Vegetarianism* and became convinced. He organized a vegetarian club and met people with theosophical and altruistic interests. His first reading of the *Bhagavad Gita* was in Edwin Arnold's poetic translation *The Song Celestial*. This Hindu scripture and the Sermon on the Mount later became his bibles and spiritual guidebooks. He memorized the *Gita* during his daily toothbrushing and often recited its original Sanskrit at his prayer meetings.

When Gandhi returned to India in 1891 his mother had died, and he was not successful at breaking into the legal profession due to his shyness. So he took the opportunity of representing an Indian firm in Natal, South Africa for a year. South Africa, which is still notorious for racial discrimination, gave Gandhi the insults which awakened his social conscience. He refused to remove his turban in court; he was thrown out of a first-class railway compartment; and he was beaten for refusing to move to the footboard of a stage-coach for the sake of a European passenger. As a lawyer Gandhi did his best to discover the facts and get the parties to accept arbitration and compromise in order to settle out of court. After solving a difficult case in this way he was elated and commented, "I had learnt to find out the better side of human nature and to enter men's hearts. I realized that the true function of a lawyer was to unite parties riven asunder." He also insisted on receiving the truth from his clients, and if he found out that they had lied he dropped their cases. He believed that the lawyer's duty was to help the court discover the truth, not to try to prove the guilty innocent. At the end of the year during a farewell party before he was to sail for India, Gandhi noticed in the newspaper that a bill was being proposed that would deprive Indians of the vote. His friends urged him to stay and lead the fight for their rights in South Africa. Gandhi founded the Natal Indian Congress in 1894, and their efforts were given considerable notice by the press. When he returned from fetching his family from India in January 1897 the South Africans tried to stop him from landing by bribing and threatening the shipowner Dada Abdulla Sheth; but Dada Abdulla was Gandhi's client, and finally after a long quarantine period Gandhi was allowed to land. The waiting mob recognized Gandhi, and some whites began to hit his face and body until the Police Superintendent's wife came to his rescue. The mob threatened to lynch him, but Gandhi escaped in a disguise. Later he refused to prosecute anyone, holding to the principle of self-restraint in regard to a personal wrong; besides, it had been the community leaders and the Natal government who caused the problem. Nevertheless Gandhi felt it his duty to support the British during the Boer War which he did by organizing and leading an Indian Ambulance Corps to nurse the wounded on the battlefield. Even this effort was somewhat delayed by race prejudice, but when three hundred free Indians and eight hundred indentured servants volunteered, the whites were impressed. Gandhi ended up spending twenty years in South Africa. He experimented with celibacy during his thirties, and in 1906 took the Brahmacharya vow for the rest of his life.

The first use of civil disobedience on a mass scale came in September 1906. The Transvaal government wanted to register the entire Indian population. The Indians held a mass meeting in the Imperial Theatre of Johannesburg; they were angry at the humiliating ordinance, and some threatened a violent response if put to the test. However, they decided as a group to refuse to comply with the registration provisions; there was complete unanimity. Yet Gandhi suggested that they take a pledge in the name of God; even though they were Hindus and Moslems they all believed in one and the same God. Every one of the nearly three thousand Indians present took the solemn pledge. Gandhi decided to call this technique of refusing to submit to injustice *"Satyagraha"* which means literally "holding to the truth." One week after the pledge Asiatic women were excused from having to register. When the Transvaal government finally put the Asiatic Registration Act into effect in 1907, Gandhi and several other Indians were arrested. He was given only two months without hard labor, and he spent the time reading. Yet during his life Gandhi would spend a total of more than six and a half years in jail. Gandhi was called to meet with General Jan Christiaan Smuts, and they agreed on a compromise. Gandhi declared to his followers that a Satyagrahi must be fearless and always trust his opponent, "for an implicit trust in human nature is the very essence of his creed." Satyagraha uncovers hidden motives and reveals the truth; even if it results in the opponent's falseness, the wrong will be more sharply felt and will be more clearly seen, and we must continually give him the opportunity to be true. While reading in jail Gandhi discovered Thoreau's "Civil Disobedience" and the works of Tolstoy. He was "overwhelmed" by *The Kingdom of God is Within You* and "began to realize more and more the infinite possibilities of universal love."

The protest movement for Indian rights in South Africa continued to grow; at one point out of the 13,000 Indians in the province 2,500 Indians were in jail, while 6,000 had fled Transvaal. In being civil to the opponents during the disobedience Gandhi developed the use of *ahimsa,* which means "non-hurting" and is usually translated "nonviolence." Gandhi followed the precept "Hate the sin and not the sinner." Since we are all one spiritually, to hurt or attack another person is to attack oneself. Though we may attack an unjust system, we must always love the persons involved. Thus "ahimsa is the basis of the search for truth."

Gandhi was also attracted to the simple agricultural life. He started two rural communes for Satyagrahis — Phoenix Farm and Tolstoy Farm. He wrote and edited the journal *Indian Opinion* to elucidate the principles and practice of Satyagraha. Three issues brought the quest for Indian rights in South Africa to a crisis — the tax on ex-serfs, the ban on Asiatic immigrants, and the invalidating of all but Christian marriages. In November 1913 Gandhi led a march of over two thousand people. Gandhi was arrested and released on bail, arrested again and released, and arrested once more all within four days. He was sentenced to three months' hard labor, but the strikes and demonstrations went on with about 50,000 indentured laborers on strike and thousands of free Indians in prison. The Christian missionary Charles F. Andrews donated all his money to the movement. Gandhi and the other leaders were released and announced another march. However, Gandhi refused to take advantage of a railway strike by white employees and called off the march in spite of Smut's broken pledge in 1908. "Forgiveness is the ornament of the brave," Gandhi explained. Finally by negotiation the issues were resolved. All marriages regardless of religion were valid; the tax on indentured laborers was cancelled including arrears; and Indians were allowed to move more freely. Gandhi summarized the power of the Satyagraha method and prophesied how it could transform modern civilization. "It is a force which, if it became universal, would revolutionize social ideals and do away with despotisms and the ever-growing militarism under which the nations of the West are groaning and are being almost crushed to death, and which fairly promises to overwhelm even the nations of the East." Smuts expressed his respect for Gandhi and his gentle but powerful methods which had made him realize that the law had to be repealed.

Meanwhile India was still suffering under British colonial rule. In 1909 Gandhi had written *Hind Swaraj* which means "Indian Self-Rule." In this diatribe against the corruption of Western civilization Gandhi suggests that India can gain its independence by nonviolent means and self-reliance. He rejects brute force and its oppression and declares that soul force or love is what keeps people together in peace and harmony. History ignores the peaceful qualities but takes note of the interruptions and violations which disrupt civilization. Gandhi returned to India in 1915 and again supported the British during the First World War by raising and leading an ambulance corps.

The great poet Rabindranath Tagore gave Gandhi the title "Mahatma" meaning "Great Soul," and Gandhi founded the Satyagraha Ashram for his family and co-workers near the textile city of Ahmedabad. When a family of untouchables asked to live in the ashram, Gandhi admitted them. Orthodox Hindus believed this polluted them. Funds ran out, and Gandhi was ready to live in the untouchable slums if necessary, but an anonymous benefactor donated enough money to last a year. To help change people's attitudes about these unfortunate pariahs, Gandhi renamed them "Harijans" or "Children of God." Later he called his weekly magazine *Harijan* also.

In 1917 Gandhi helped the indigo sharecroppers of Champaran throw off the unfair exploitation of their landlords. He was arrested, but the officials soon realized that the Mahatma was the only one who could control the crowds. Reforms were won again by civil disobedience, this time in India. The textile workers of Ahmedabad were also economically oppressed. Gandhi suggested a strike, and when the workers were weakening in their resolve he went on a fast to encourage them to continue the strike. Gandhi explained that he did not fast to coerce the opponent but to strengthen or reform those who loved him. He did not believe in fasting for higher wages, but he fasted so that the workers would accept the system of arbitration to resolve the conflict, which they did.

Gandhi's first challenge to the British government in India was in response to the arbitrary powers of the Rowlatt Act in 1919. India had cooperated with Britain during the war, and instead of receiving Dominion Status civil liberties were being curtailed. Guided by a dream or inner experience Gandhi decided to call for a one-day hartal or general strike on all economic activity. Many signed the Satyagraha pledge, and Gandhi suggested making "a continuous and persistent effort to return good for evil." However, the philosophy was not well understood by the masses, and violence erupted in various places. The Mahatma repented declaring he had made "a Himalayan miscalculation," and he called off the campaign. In one infamous incident General Dyer had ordered his soldiers to fire into a crowd, wounding 1,137 and killing 379. The Hunter Report indicated that he was less concerned with dispersing the crowd and more intent on "producing a sufficient moral effect from a military point of view." Another general made the statement: "Force is the only thing that an Asiatic has any respect for." The report concluded that the moral effect was quite opposite from the one intended.

Gandhi founded and published two weeklies without advertisements — *Young India* in English and *Navajivan* in Gujarati. In 1920 Gandhi initiated a nation-wide campaign of non-cooperation with the British government, which for the peasant meant non-payment of taxes and no buying of liquor since the government gained revenue from its sale. Gandhi traveled throughout India addressing mass meetings. He urged people to spin their own cloth and designed a Congress flag with a spinning wheel in the center. By January 1922 thirty thousand

Indians had been jailed for civil disobedience. Some nationalist patriots urged revolution, but Gandhi would never forsake nonviolence. Gandhi decided to try mass civil disobedience in Bardoli, a county of 87,000, but news of how an Indian mob had murdered some constables reached him. Although it was eight hundred miles from Bardoli, he once again canceled the campaign, this time before it had started. In March the British Viceroy ordered Gandhi's arrest. This was the only time that the British allowed him a trial. He made no apology and suggested the highest penalty "for what in law is a deliberate crime and what appears to me to be the highest duty of a citizen." Gandhi explained, "In my opinion, non-cooperation with evil is as much a duty as is cooperation with good." The judge sentenced him to six years and hoped the government would reduce the term. He was in fact released after twenty-two months when he had an appendectomy.

Perhaps the greatest block to Indian unity and self-government was the conflict between Hindus and Moslems. In 1924 Gandhi went on a twenty-one day fast to bridge this strife. He pleaded for unity in diversity, religious tolerance, and love for one another.

During the late 1920s Gandhi wrote an autobiography which he called his experiments with truth; it is quite candid and humble in the way he examines his faults and his efforts to overcome them. In his speeches he pointed out his five-point program on the fingers of his hand: equality for untouchables, spinning, no alcohol or drugs, Hindu-Moslem friendship, and equality for women. They were all connected to the wrist which stood for nonviolence. Finally in 1928 he announced a Satyagraha campaign in Bardoli against a 22% increase in British-imposed taxes. Refusing to pay taxes the people had their possessions confiscated and some were driven off their land, but they remained nonviolent. It lasted several months, and hundreds were arrested. Finally the government gave in and agreed to cancel the tax increase, release all prisoners, and return confiscated land and property; the peasants agreed to pay their taxes at the previous rate.

The Indian Congress wanted self-government and considered war for independence. Gandhi naturally refused to support a war but declared that if India was not free under Dominion Status by the end of 1929, then he would demand independence. Consequently in 1930 he informed the Viceroy that civil disobedience would begin on March 11. "My ambition is no less than to convert the British people through nonviolence, and thus make them see the wrong they have done to India. I do not seek to harm your people." Gandhi decided to disobey the Salt Laws which forbade Indians from making their own salt; this British monopoly especially struck at the poor. Beginning with seventy-eight members of his ashram Gandhi led a two-hundred mile march to the sea over twenty-four days. Thousands had gathered at the start, and several thousands joined them on the march. First Gandhi and then others all along the seacoast gathered some salt water in pans to dry it. In Bombay the Congress had pans on the roof; 60,000 people assembled, and hundreds were arrested. At Karachi where 50,000 watched the salt being made, the crowd was so thick that the police could make no arrests. The jails were filled with at least 60,000 offenders. Amazingly enough there was practically no violence at all; the people did not want Gandhi to cancel the movement. Gandhi was arrested before he could invade the Dharasana Salt Works, but his friend Mrs. Sarojini Naidu led 2,500 volunteers and warned them not to resist the blows of the police. According to an eye-witness account by the reporter Webb Miller, they continued to march in until beaten down with steel-shod lathis by the four hundred police, but they did not try to fight back. Tagore declared that Europe had lost her moral prestige in Asia. Soon more than 100,000 Indians were in prison, including almost all the leaders.

Gandhi was called to a meeting with Viceroy Irwin in 1931, and they came to an agreement in March. Civil disobedience was called off; prisoners were released; salt manufacture was permitted on the coast; and Congress leaders would attend the next Round Table Conference in London. Gandhi traveled to London where he met Charlie Chaplin, George Bernard Shaw, and Maria Montessori among others. On radio to the United

States he spoke of a way better than brute force more consistent with human dignity. In discussing relations with the British he said he did not want isolated independence but voluntary interdependence based on love.

While in prison in 1932 Gandhi went on a fast on behalf of the Harijans because they had been given a separate electorate. It was to be a "fast unto death" unless he could awaken the Hindu conscience. The issue was resolved, and even Hindu temples were opened to untouchables for the first time. The next year Gandhi went on a twenty-one day fast for purification, and British officials, afraid he might die, released him from prison. Gandhi announced that he would not engage in civil disobedience until his sentence was completed.

By the time the second world war was approaching Gandhi had been confirmed in his pacifist principles. He pointed out how Abyssinia could have used nonviolence against Mussolini, and he recommended it to the Czechs and China. "If it is brave, as it is, to die to a man fighting against odds, it is braver still to refuse to fight and yet to refuse to yield to the usurper." As early as 1938 he exhorted the Jews to stand up for their rights and die if necessary as martyrs. "A degrading manhunt can be turned into a calm and determined stand offered by unarmed men and women possessing the strength given to them by Jehovah." Gandhi even recommended to the British nonviolent methods of fighting Hitler; no longer could he support any kind of war or killing. He decided on mass Satyagraha in defiance of the ban on propaganda against the war. Gandhi promised Congress he would stay out of jail, but 23,223 others were arrested including Vinoba Bhave, Nehru, and Patel. In 1942 Gandhi suggested ways to resist the Japanese nonviolently. He sent an appeal to the Japanese people for the sake of "world federation and brotherhood without which there can be no hope for humanity."

However, Gandhi continued to preach a nonviolent revolution for India, and in 1942 he and other leaders were arrested. He decided to fast again; he barely survived. When the war ended he asserted the need for "a real peace based on the freedom and equality of all races and nations." In his last years he became more of a socialist. He said, "Violence is bred by inequality, nonviolence by equality." He went on a pilgrimage to Noakhali to help the poor. Independence for India was now imminent, but Jinnah the Moslem leader was holding out for the creation of a separate state of Pakistan. Gandhi prayed for unity and tolerance, and he even read from the Koran at his prayer meetings. Hindus attacked him because they thought he was partial to Moslems, and Moslems demanded he let them have Pakistan. Gandhi went to Calcutta to calm the Hindu-Moslem strife and violence. Once more he fasted until the community leaders signed a pledge to keep the peace; before they signed he warned them that if they broke their word he would fast until he died. His last fast in January 1948 also did much to heal the conflicts between the Hindus and the Moslems over the division into two countries which left minorities in both nations. Although this religious hatred saddened Gandhi, India had gained her independence on August 15, 1947 accomplishing the greatest nonviolent revolution in the history of the world. Finally Gandhi was assassinated by an outraged Hindu on January 30, 1948 at a prayer meeting; with his last breath the Mahatma chanted the name of God.

Albert Einstein declared that Gandhi showed how someone could win allegiance, "not merely by the cunning game of political fraud and trickery, but through the living example of a morally exalted way of life." Einstein considered Gandhi to be the most enlightened statesman of their time, and he predicted, "The problem of bringing peace to the world on a supranational basis will be solved only by employing Gandhi's method on a large scale." The Encyclopaedia Britannica summarizes Gandhi's significance with the statement, "He was the catalyst if not the initiator of three of the major revolutions of the 20th century: the revolutions against colonialism, racism, and violence." What was his philosophy of nonviolent soul-force, and what instructions did he give in the use of these methods?

"Satyagraha" means literally holding on to the Truth. The Hindu understanding of *Sat* is more than conceptual truth but means also being, existence, reality; ultimately we realize that our spiritual beingness is the essence of Truth as a reality greater than any concept of the mind. Thus the term "soul-force" conveys the idea of employing our spiritual energies. For Gandhi this Truth or spiritual reality is the goal, and the means to the goal must be as pure and loving as possible. Ahimsa therefore is the way of acting without hurting anyone or inflicting oneself against another spiritual being. We may hate an injustice for the harm that it brings to people, but we must always love all the people involved out of respect for human dignity. Satyagraha attempts to awaken an awareness of the truth about the injustice in the perpetrators, and by ahimsa this is done without hurting them. Since humans are subject to error and we cannot be sure we are judging accurately, we must refrain from punishing. Thus ahimsa is an essential safeguard in the quest for truth and justice.

Gandhi explains that Satyagraha is not a method of the weak, like passive resistance, but "a weapon of the strong and excludes the use of violence in any shape or form." Satyagraha is insisting on the truth and can be offered in relation to one's family, rulers, fellow citizens, or even the whole world. Gandhi elucidates three necessary conditions for its success: "1) The Satyagrahi should not have any hatred in his heart against the opponent. 2) The issue must be true and substantial. 3) The Satyagrahi must be prepared to suffer till the end for his cause." Gandhi emphasized self-suffering rather than inflicting suffering on others. By undergoing suffering to reveal the injustice the Satyagrahi strives to reach the consciences of people. Satyagraha does not try to coerce anyone but rather to convert by persuasion, to reach the reason through the heart. Satyagraha appeals to intelligent public opinion for reform. In the political field the struggle on behalf of the people leads to the challenging of unjust governments or laws by means of non-cooperation or civil disobedience. When petitions and other remedies fail, then a Satyagrahi may break an unjust law and willingly suffer the penalty in order to call attention to the injustice. However, he does not hide or try to escape from the law like a criminal, rather he openly and civilly disobeys the law as a protest, fully expecting to be punished. In *Hind Swaraj* Gandhi wrote, "It is contrary to our manhood if we obey laws repugnant to our conscience." By eliminating violence Satyagraha gives the opponent the same rights and liberties. Satyagraha requires self-discipline, self-control, and self-purification, and Satyagrahis must always make the distinction between the evil and the evil-doer. They must overcome evil with good, hatred with love, anger with patience, untruth with truth, and violence with ahimsa. This takes a perfect person for complete success, and therefore training and education are essential to even make it workable. Gandhi emphasizes that every child "should know what the soul is, what truth is, what love is, what powers are latent in the soul." Both men and women, and even children, may participate, and it demands the courage that comes from spiritual strength and the power of love. Surely it takes more courage to face the weapons of death without fighting than it does to fight and kill. From his experience Gandhi believed that those who wished to serve their country through Satyagraha should "observe perfect chastity, adopt poverty, follow truth, and cultivate fearlessness." It is through fearlessness that we can have the courage to renounce all harmful weapons, filling and surrounding ourselves with the spiritual protection of a loving and peaceful consciousness.

Gandhi elucidated specific guidelines for Satyagraha and civil disobedience. A Satyagrahi will not harbor anger but will suffer the opponent's anger and assaults without retaliating. However, he or she will not submit out of fear of punishment nor obey any order given in anger. Satyagrahis will voluntarily and civilly submit to arrest and will not resist the confiscation of their property; but if a civil resister has the property of another as a trustee, he will refuse to surrender it, holding on to it at the cost of his life. Satyagrahis will not insult or curse their opponents nor participate in shouted cries which are contrary to the spirit of love (ahimsa). Civil resisters will not salute the flag of the government against which they are protesting, but they will not insult it or the government officials. In fact they will protect officials from assault even at the risk of life.

Non-cooperation is a comprehensive policy used by people when they can no longer in good conscience participate in or support a government that has become oppressive, unjust, and violent. Although Satyagrahis do not attack the wrong-doer, it is their responsibility not to promote or support the wrong actions.

Thus non-cooperators withdraw from government positions, renounce government programs and services, and refuse to pay taxes to the offending government. While challenging the power of the state in this way non-cooperators have the opportunity to learn greater self-reliance. Gandhi held that non-cooperation with an unjust government was not only an inherent right but as much a duty as is cooperation with a just government.

Ahimsa or nonviolence is absolutely essential to Gandhi's civil disobedience. Satyagrahis were expected to give their lives in efforts to quell violence if it erupted. Gandhi interpreted ahimsa broadly as refraining from anything at all harmful. "The principle of ahimsa is hurt by every evil thought, by undue haste, by lying, by hatred, by wishing ill to anybody. It is also violated by our holding on to what the world needs." Thus even greed and avarice can violate ahimsa. Nonviolence has a great spiritual power, but the slightest use of violence can taint a just cause. The strength is not physical but comes from the spiritual will. The following is Gandhi's summary of the implications of nonviolence:

1) Nonviolence is the law of the human race and is infinitely greater than and superior to brute force.
2) In the last resort it does not avail to those who do not possess a living faith in the God of Love.
3) Nonviolence affords the fullest protection to one's self-respect and sense of honour, but not always to possession of land or movable property, though its habitual practice does prove a better bulwark than the possession of armed men to defend them. Nonviolence, in the very nature of things, is of no assistance in the defense of ill-gotten gains and immoral acts.
4) Individuals or nations who would practice nonviolence must be prepared to sacrifice (nations to the last man) their all except honour. It is, therefore, inconsistent with the possession of other people's countries, i.e., modern imperialism, which is frankly based on force for its defense.
5) Nonviolence is a power which can be wielded equally by all — children, young men and women or grown-up people, provided they have a living faith in the God of

Love and have therefore equal love for all mankind. When nonviolence is accepted as the law of life it must pervade the whole being and not be applied to isolated acts.
6) It is a profound error to suppose that whilst the law is good enough for individuals it is not for masses of mankind.

Gandhi's struggle was so overwhelming and significant, because he challenged the institutional violence of the modern state. He not only recommended refusing military service but also refusing to pay taxes to a militarized state. In addition to citizens' non-cooperating with an evil government, a neutral country also has the obligation to refuse to support or assist a military state or aggressor. Gandhi suggested a nonviolent army that could engage in constructive activities, lessen tensions, and sacrifice their lives to calm mobs and end riots. The qualifications for such a peace brigade would be complete faith in and adherence to nonviolence, equal respect for all religions, personal service and good human relations with the community, integrity and impartiality, and anticipation of brooding conflicts. The cost of training and equipping such a peace brigade would be practically nothing compared to the expenses of the modern military establishment. Gandhi envisioned a nonviolent state which would protect itself by not cooperating with any aggressor. Gandhi was concerned that the democracies would adopt the forceful methods of the fascists; but true democracy must ultimately be nonviolent, for violence is an obvious restriction of liberty. In 1946 Gandhi asserted, "Democracy to be true should cease to rely upon the army for anything whatsoever. It will be a poor democracy that depends for its existence on military assistance. Military force interferes with the free growth of the mind. It smothers the soul of man." He criticized America for its treatment of the Negro. Gandhi observed that armaments are used for greedy exploitation and that the competition and desire for material possessions and the Great Power's imperialistic designs are the biggest blocks to world peace. Also they must shed their fear of destruction; then by disarmament peace can be attained. Gandhi warned, "If the mad race for armaments continues, it is bound to result in a slaughter such as has never occurred in history. If there is a victor left, the very victory will be a living death for the nation that emerges victorious. There is no escape from the impending doom save through a bold and unconditional acceptance of the nonviolent method with all its glorious implications." Gandhi urged us to go beyond family and country to consider the good of the world, and he recommended a world governing body which would recognize the equal independence of each nation. He once said, "The golden way is to be friends with the world and to regard the whole human family as one."

15

Woodrow Wilson and the League of Nations

"Friendship is the only cement
that will ever hold the world together."

Woodrow Wilson

"Interest does not bind men together:
interest separates men.
There is only one thing that can bind men together,
and that is common devotion to right."

Woodrow Wilson

"What we seek is the reign of law,
based upon the consent of the governed,
and sustained by the organized opinion of mankind."

Woodrow Wilson

"President Wilson had come to Europe
with a program of peace for all men.
His ideal was a very high one,
but it involved great difficulties,
owing to these century-old hatreds between some races."

Georges Clemenceau

"Political liberty can exist only when there is peace.
Social reform can take place only when there is peace."

Woodrow Wilson

The tragic story of the League of Nations centers around the man who conceived it and offered it to the world, who developed its charter and bore the pains of its formulation at the Peace Conference in France, and who broke down in exhaustion when his own nation, the United States, refused to ratify it in the Senate. Thomas Woodrow Wilson was born December 28, 1856 in Staunton, Virginia. His father was a Presbyterian minister, and Woodrow was a deeply religious man throughout his life. He was fascinated by politics and longed to be a statesman like England's Prime Minister Gladstone. He wrote steveral books on government and taught political economy at Princeton University. As an educational reformer he was unanimously chosen president of Princeton in 1902. Wilson emphasized broad liberal studies more than specialization and mere preparation for a career. In 1910 the Democratic Party nominated him for governor of New Jersey, and his persuasive expression of progressive principles swept him to victory. His liberal reforms were successful, and in 1912 he won the Democratic presidential nomination and then a popular plurality over the divided Republicans and Theodore Roosevelt's Progressive Party. He offered "New Freedom" and set out to break up the privileges of trusts and tariffs; he championed the worker's right to overtime pay beyond an eight-hour day. However, his greatest challenges were to be in foreign policy after the outbreak of the World War in 1914.

From the close of the Napoleonic wars and the Congress of Vienna in 1815 some popular support for peace societies which were founded at that time and a concern for international law enabled national leaders to solve many of their differences by means of arbitration. Between 1815 and 1900, of the two hundred cases in which States agreed to arbitration, not a single case led to a war. However, the States had not pledged that they would submit to arbitration in every international conflict. In 1890 the United States and ten other American republics signed a Pan American Treaty of Arbitration, but it was not ratified. In 1899 and again in 1907 the Russian Czar Nicolas II called a conference at The Hague to discuss limitation of arms and peaceful methods to settle international disputes. A "Permanent Court of Arbitration" was set up which could be used to resolve differences, and in fact three dangerous conflicts between large powers were settled in this manner. Theodore Roosevelt submitted a dispute with Mexico to arbitration, and in 1903 Britain and France signed a treaty. Roosevelt followed their example and signed arbitration treaties with France, Germany, Portugal, and Switzerland. He was negotiating with Great Britain, Italy, Mexico, Russia, Japan, and others when the Senate led by Henry Cabot Lodge insisted on approving each treaty. T. R. felt this undercut his efforts and therefore abandoned them. Roosevelt supported arbitration and arms limitation at the second Hague Conference. While receiving the Nobel Peace Prize in 1910 he spoke of a League of Peace which the great powers could form "not only to keep the peace among themselves, but to prevent, by force if necessary, its being broken by others." The problem with The Hague approach, he believed, was that it lacked an effective executive police power. Roosevelt stated concisely, "Each nation must keep well prepared to defend itself until the establishment of some form of international police power, competent and willing to prevent violence as between nations. As things are now, such power to command peace throughout the world could best be assured by some combination between those great nations which sincerely desire peace and have no thought of themselves of committing aggressions." Roosevelt concluded that the statesman who could bring this about would have the gratitude of all mankind.

In the spring of 1914 President Wilson sent his close friend and advisor, Colonel House, to Europe as an unofficial ambassador for peace. House met with German officials and the Kaiser explaining that with the community of interests between England, Germany, and the United States they could together maintain the peace of the world. However, England was concerned about Germany's growing navy. House went to Paris and then London where he conferred with Edward Grey about negotiating with Germany. Even after the assassination of Archduke Ferdinand, the event which precipitated the war, House returned to Berlin and appealed to the Kaiser through a letter that England, France, and Germany could settle their differences peacefully. Many years later the Kaiser admitted that the mediation offer by Wilson and House had almost prevented the war. However, the German militarists were intent on fighting, and the war broke out with Austria leading the way. President Wilson on August 19 declared that the United States was neutral, and he requested that the American people be impartial. In January 1915 Wilson again sent House to Europe on a peace mission, hoping to get a parley started to discover possible terms and conditions of peace.

In England a League of Nations Society was founded in May 1915, and the idea of a League was supported publicly by Grey and Asquith. In the United States numerous branches of the League to Enforce Peace sprang up around the country. On May 27, 1916 this group, supported by ex-President William H. Taft, heard speeches by President Wilson and the Republican Senator Henry Cabot Lodge. Lodge was wary of forming entangling alliances, about which Washington had warned America, but this he felt should not preclude joining with other civilized nations to diminish war and encourage peace. In fact the Senator stated strongly, "We must find some way in which the united forces of the nations could be put behind the cause of peace and law." In his speech Wilson also declared, "The nations of the world must in some way band themselves together to see that that right prevails as against any sort of selfish aggression." Civilization is not yet firmly established until nations are governed by the same code of conduct that we demand of individuals. He outlined three fundamental principles: first, that every people has the right to choose their sovereignty; second, that small nations as well as large ones ought to have the guarantee of territorial integrity; and third, that the world and the rights of its people and nations ought to be protected from disturbing aggression. He proposed that the United States initiate a movement for peace calling for a "universal association of the nations" to maintain security of the above principles with the help of world opinion.

While speaking to West Point graduates that year Wilson contrasted the spirit of militarism to the citizen spirit, and asserted that in the United States the civilian spirit is intended to dominate the military, which is why the President, a civilian authority, is commander-in-chief of all forces. In September Wilson was renominated by the Democratic Party, and in his acceptance speech he discussed world peace. America must contribute to a just and settled peace, because no longer can any nation remain wholly apart from world turmoil. Again he appealed to world opinion to establish joint guarantees for peace and justice in a spirit of friendship. Wilson's re-election was promoted under the slogan "He kept us out of war," and he managed to win a narrow victory.

In January 1917 the Germans decided to pursue unrestricted submarine warfare. Wilson was trying to get the western allies and central powers to negotiate peace with each other, and he was not informed of the Germans' change in policy when he delivered his great "Peace without Victory" speech on January 22. This was the first time a President had appeared alone before the Senate since George Washington vowed never to return there. Wilson expressed his hope that peace could be negotiated soon, and he was convinced that after the war an international concert of power must prevent war. He offered the United States Government in its tradition of upholding liberty to serve in using its authority and power to guarantee peace and justice throughout the world by means of a League for Peace. The President wanted to indicate the conditions upon which the United States could enter into this process. First the war must be ended, and by a treaty of peace that will be universally approved and guaranteed by a universal covenant, which must include the peoples of the New World. The organized force of mankind protecting the peace must be greater than any nation or probable combination of nations. Wilson did not believe that the war should end in a new balance of power but rather in a just and organized common peace, for no one can guarantee the stability of a balance of power. Neither side really intends to crush the other; therefore it must be a peace without victory so that the victor will not impose intolerable sacrifices which result in resentment and probably future hostilities. Equality of nations is the right attitude for a lasting peace as well as a just settlement regarding territory and national allegiance. Equality of nations means a respect for the rights of small nations based upon the common strength of the concert of nations, not upon individual strength. A deeper principle yet is that "governments derive all their just powers from the consent of the governed, and that no right anywhere exists to hand peoples about from sovereignty to sovereignty as if they were property. That henceforth inviolable security of life, of worship, and of industrial and social development should be guaranteed to all peoples." Peace can only be stable with justice and freedom; otherwise the spirit rebels. Wilson asserted the importance of freedom of the seas and also the need to limit navies and armies. Wilson felt that he was speaking "for liberals and friends of humanity in every nation ... for the silent mass of mankind." He suggested that the American principles of the Monroe Doctrine should be extended throughout the world so that "every people should be left free to determine its own polity, its own way of development, unhindered, unthreatened, unafraid." These principles of self-determination, freedom, and protection from aggression "are the principles of mankind and must prevail."

Wilson struggled to keep America out of the war, but when the Germans announced submarine warfare even against neutral shipping he immediately broke diplomatic relations with Germany. American intelligence reports indicated that Germany was trying to form an alliance with Mexico against the United States. Wilson had considered entry into the war a crime against civilization, and he loathed the implications. Privately he said, "It would mean that we would lose our heads along with the rest and stop weighing right and wrong. It would mean that a majority of people in this hemisphere would go war mad, quit thinking, and devote their energies to destruction." However, in March several U.S. ships were attacked, and the President decided to propose a declaration of war to the Congress on April 2. He appealed to international law and the freedom of the seas. Because of the loss of noncombatants' lives he interpreted the German submarine warfare against commerce as a "warfare against mankind." He did not recommend revenge or the victorious assertion of physical might as motives for action but rather the vindication of human right and a refusal to submit to wrongs. Therefore since the Imperial German Government was at war with the United States, they must accept the belligerent status thrust upon them. Wilson clearly stated his purpose for America's role, "Our object is to vindicate the principles of peace and justice in the life of the world as against selfish and autocratic power and to set up amongst the really free and self-governed peoples of the world such a concert of purpose and of action as will henceforth insure the observance of those principles." He declared that a new age was beginning in which nations and governments must be held to the same standards of conduct and responsibility as the individual citizens of civilized states. He indicated that America had no animosity toward the German people, and he explained that small groups of ambitious men were using those people as pawns under the veil of the private courts of a privileged class. Wilson believed that peace could only be maintained by a partnership of democratic nations; autocratic governments cannot be trusted. Therefore Americans must fight for the liberation of the world's people, including the German peoples. "The world must be made safe for democracy." Peace must be founded on political liberty. President Wilson disavowed any desire for conquest or dominion; America was to be merely one of the champions of mankind's rights. Wilson's speech was greeted with wildly enthusiastic applause; later he thought how strange it was to hear applause for a message that meant death for many young men.

The United States was involved in the World War, but it would be six months before many soldiers would be fighting in France. That summer President Wilson appointed an Inquiry of several distinguished experts to gather information on Europe's oppressed peoples, international business, international law, proposals for a peace-keeping organization, and ideas on repairing the war damage in Belgium and France. Wilson prophetically warned, "What we are seeking is a basis that will be fair to all and which will nowhere plant the seeds of such jealousy and discontent and restraint of development as would certainly breed future wars."

Utilizing this research by experts Wilson formulated the war aims and peace suggestions of the United States and presented them before Congress on January 8, 1918 as his famous Fourteen Points. He reiterated that the United States was seeking only a peaceful world that is safe for self-governing nations. His specific points may be summarized as follows: 1) "open covenants of peace, openly arrived at" — no secret treaties; 2) free navigation of the seas outside territorial waters; 3) equality of trade and removal of economic barriers; 4) "adequate guarantees given and taken that national armaments will be reduced to the lowest point consistent with domestic safety;" 5) impartial adjustment of all colonial claims weighing equally the interests of the populations with the claims of governments; 6) evacuation of Russian territory and the opportunity for Russians to choose their own institutions, and aid according to their needs and desires; 7) evacuation and restoration of Belgium under her own sovereignty; 8) liberation and restoration of invaded French territory and the return of Alsace-Lorraine to France, correcting the wrong of 1871; 9) "a readjustment of the frontiers of Italy should be effected along clearly recognizable lines of nationality;" 10) the peoples of Austria-Hungary should be freely allowed autonomous development; 11) Rumania, Serbia, and Montenegro should be evacuated and restored, and the Balkan states ought to be established along lines of allegiance and nationality with international guarantees of independence and territorial integrity, with access to the sea for Serbia; 12) Turkey itself should have secure sovereignty, but other nationalities should be freed of Turkish rule and be assured of autonomous development, and the Dardanelles should be open to all ships and commerce under international guarantees; 13) an independent Poland should include territories of Polish populations, have access to the sea and guaranteed territorial integrity; and 14) "a general association of nations must be formed under specific covenants for the purpose of affording mutual guarantees of political independence and territorial integrity to great and small states alike." The President then declared that the United States was willing to fight for these principles to secure liberty and safety for all peoples under international justice. Germany was to be allowed her fair and equal place among the nations, and Wilson requested negotiation with representatives of the majority of German people rather than the military party and imperialists.

These Fourteen Points were adopted by the Allied statesmen as a basis for the peace. Responses to this speech soon came from representatives of Germany and Austria. These replies by Count von Hertling and Count Czernin were answered by Wilson in a speech on February 11; he was especially critical of the German Chancellor von Hertling. Peace must be established justly in view of world opinion and not involving militarily only the separate states that are most powerful. Wilson also pointed out that there were to be no annexations, no punitive damages, no arbitrary handing of people about by antagonists, but respect for national aspirations and self-determination.

Wilson again summarized the great ideals America was fighting for in a 4th of July speech at Mount Vernon. Over a million American men had already been shipped to France. The four goals he stated were: 1) destruction of every arbitrary power that disturbs the world's peace; 2) settlement of political and economic questions with the consent of those involved, not according to the material interests of other nations; 3) consent of all nations to live under common law and mutual respect for justice; and 4) establishment of a peace organization of the free nations' combined power to check violations of peace and justice according to the tribunal of international opinion to which all must submit.

By the end of summer 1918 the Central Powers were breaking up, and on September 27 Wilson appealed to the peoples of those countries by suggesting more specific peace proposals. Once more he emphasized that right must be made superior to might. The idea of a League of Nations was beginning to take a more definite shape. Each government must be willing to pay the price necessary to achieve impartial justice, to be made effective by the instrumentality of a League of Nations. The constitution of the League of Nations must be a part of the peace settlement, for if it preceded peace it would be confined to the nations allied against a common enemy, and if it followed the peace settlement it could not guarantee the peace terms. Wilson then outlined five particulars: 1) impartial justice means no discrimination or favoritism between peoples; 2) no special interest of a single nation should infringe upon the common interest of all; 3) "there can be no leagues or alliances or special covenants and understandings within the general and common family of the League of Nations;" 4) there can be no selfish economic combinations or boycotts except as "may be vested in the League of Nations itself as a means of discipline and control;" and 5) "all international agreements and treaties of every kind must be made known in their entirety to the rest of the world."

On October 6 the German government requested an armistice; President Wilson sent a reply declaring that the armies of the

Central Powers must withdraw immediately from all invaded territory. A German response dodged the issue of evacuation, and therefore another message clarifying the military situation was sent through the Secretary of State. On October 25 Wilson made perhaps one of his worst political mistakes when he requested the election of a Democratic majority in Congress in order to indicate to the world American support of the President's leadership. This intrusion of party politics into non-partisan foreign affairs was deeply resented by Republicans and in fact backfired against Wilson, as the Republicans won both houses. Meanwhile the Germans had agreed to disarm and relinquish the monarchical military leadership and wanted a peace according to the points made in Wilson's speeches. Austria-Hungary also accepted the President's declarations and recognized the rights of the Czecho-Slovaks and the Jugo-Slavs. The Allied Governments agreed to accept the Fourteen Points and the subsequent addresses with one reservation by Great Britain on freedom of the seas. Poland and Germany each announced themselves as republics. Finally on November 11 German representatives signed the Armistice Agreement at Marshall Foch's headquarters. The Germans had agreed to an almost total surrender and to the payment of reparations. On the same day, President Wilson read the Armistice Agreement to Congress and promised food and relief to a suffering Europe. He pointed out the disorder in Russia and the folly of attempting conquest by the force of arms, and he asserted, "The nations that have learned the discipline of freedom and that have settled with self-possession to its ordered practice are now about to make conquest of the world by the sheer power of example of friendly helpfulness." America must hold the light for the peoples who were just then coming into their freedom. A peace must be established that will define their places among the nations and protect their security.

Wilson decided to attend the Peace Conference in France with a select group of experts, such as geographers, ethnologists, and economists, whom he told, "Tell me what is right, and I'll fight for it." Unfortunately he did not invite anyone from the Senate to attend, which later was to cause irreconcilable problems. In

Europe Wilson was enthusiastically greeted by thousands of cheering people almost as a messiah. In London on December 30 he observed, "Never before in the history of the world, I believe, has there been such a keen international consciousness as there is now." On the same day in Manchester he spoke of America's desire for peace in the world, not merely a balance of power or peace in Europe. At Rome on January 3, 1919 President Wilson explained how military force is unable to hold people together, that only friendship and good will can bind nations together. "Therefore, our task at Paris is to organize the friendship of the world, to see to it that all the moral forces that make for right and justice and liberty are united and are given a vital organization to which the peoples of the world will readily and gladly respond."

The idealistic American President who wanted only permanent peace under universal justice with no special rewards for his country faced an awesome challenge among the European old-school diplomats who were determined to gain all they could for their own national interests. Lloyd George had just been re-elected British Prime Minister under the slogan "Be tough on Germany," and Clemenceau of France was even more adamant about making Germany pay all she could and leaving her as weak as possible. The Italians and Japanese wanted control of specific territories, and secret treaties made between the Allies during the war were to emerge and confound several of Wilson's points. Against Wilson's protests the conference news was censored, and what did leak out to the press tended to be through the French newspapers controlled by their government.

Meanwhile most of Europe was in turmoil, and many military leaders wanted to grab what they could get. For this reason on January 24 Wilson published a statement warning those who would take possession of territory by force that they would be prejudicing their cause, since they were placing in doubt the justice of their claims which the Peace Conference must determine. The next day he addressed the Peace Conference, which he felt had two purposes — not only the settlements required by the war but also the secure establishment of a means for the maintaining of world peace. Wilson believed the League of Nations was necessary for both purposes. "Settlements may be temporary, but the action of the nations in the interest of peace and justice must be permanent. We can set up permanent processes. We may not be able to set up permanent decisions." Therefore the League of Nations must be made vital and continuous so that it may be ever watchful and effective. The idea for a League as an essential part of the Treaty was adopted unanimously, and a subcommittee for the drafting of a League of Nations Covenant was selected with President Wilson as chairman.

General Jan Christiaan Smuts, the leader from South Africa who had confronted Gandhi, published a pamphlet, *The League of Nations: A Practical Suggestion,* calling for a strong and active League which would not only prevent wars but also be a living, working organ of peaceful civilization. It must have general control of international affairs involving commerce, communications, and social, industrial, and labor relations. Wilson and Colonel House, the American members of the committee, managed to get together with the British delegates Smuts and Lord Cecil, who also had his own draft, to hammer out what was called Wilson's second draft, which was revised into an Anglo-American version. Although the French and Italians submitted drafts, this version was accepted as the basis for discussion. Working every night the committee of fourteen members turned out its Draft Agreement after eleven days. Wilson announced that a living thing had been born.

On January 27 Wilson suggested a solution to the problem of what to do about the German colonies. Because he felt world opinion was against annexations, the League of Nations could mandate that districts be administered by a mandatory power "with a view to the betterment of the conditions of the inhabitants" and without discriminatory economic access.

A proud President Wilson presented the League of Nations draft to the Peace Conference with an address on February 14. The League was to consist of a body of delegates, an executive council, and a permanent secretariat. Any issue of international relationship would have free discussion, for "that is the moral force of the public opinion of the world." Nevertheless if moral force did not suffice, armed force was to be in the background, but only as a last resort. The League was designed to be simple and flexible, yet a definite guarantee of peace, at least in words. Securing peace was not the only purpose of the League; it could be used for cooperation in any international matter, such as ameliorating labor conditions. All international agreements must be registered with the secretary general and openly published. Wilson believed the mandatory policy of aiding development was a great advance over annexation and exploitation. All in all Wilson felt that they had created a document that was both practical and humane, that could serve the conscience of the world. The day after the draft was accepted by the plenary session, the President departed for the United States.

In Washington Wilson met with Congressional representatives to discuss the League. By the time he returned to France in March American public opinion was insisting on four alterations. First, the Monroe Doctrine must be explicitly protected. Second, there must be a way nations could withdraw from the League. Third, domestic disputes must be exempt from League interference, including tariffs and immigration quotas. Fourth, a nation must have the right to refuse a mandate for a territory. Wilson did not feel that these provisions were necessary, but he was willing to get them put into the covenant for the sake of its acceptance. However, he had to compromise in order to do so, and thus his position on other issues was weakened.

Colonel House had been compromising on every side at the Peace talks such that when Wilson returned to Paris, he felt he had to start all over again. This caused an irreparable breach between the President and his close friend and advisor. The Allies were forcing unbearable reparations and indemnities on Germany and the defeated nations. Wilson did not consider it wise for England to retain naval supremacy or for the American and British navies to patrol the world together. Militarism on the sea is the same as on the land. He felt that power must not be vested in a single nation or combination of nations; the sea is a free highway and should be protected by a league of all the nations under international law. To fulfill one of his most important points Wilson developed a comprehensive plan for disarmament. Armaments were only to be used to preserve domestic safety and to maintain international order according to the League. Compulsory military service and the private manufacture of munitions must be abolished. Disarmament policies must be worked out after the peace settlement, be unanimously agreed upon, and have publicity to assure compliance. Although disarmament was temporarily forced upon Germany, these policies were never universally carried out. Wilson persistently argued for a new attitude of mind, for an organization of cooperation for peace which considered moral force above armed force.

Returning to the negotiations of the peace settlement Wilson faced intransigent obstacles to his principles. Several territorial arrangements had already been agreed upon by the major powers during the war in such secret agreements as the Sykes-Picot Treaty and the Treaty of London. Wilson spoke up for self-determination, and at his suggestion a commission of inquiry was sent to the Middle East to discover what the peoples' wishes were. The other powers verbally agreed but never did send their representatives. By the time the Americans went and returned with their information, the issues had been settled. The French wanted not only Alsace-Lorraine but the coal mining district of Saar and a buffer state in the Rhineland. Italy wanted not only the opposite coast of the Adriatic including Trieste which had been promised in the Treaty of London, but they also demanded the port of Fiume which represented Yugoslavia's only hope for a commercial port. England and Japan had divided up the German colonies in the Pacific Ocean, giving Japan those north of the equator and Britain those south of the equator, but Japan also wanted Shantung on the mainland. In early April Wilson became ill. He had reached the limit of his patience and requested that the oceanliner *George Washington* be prepared to take him home. The President decided to take his stand on the issue of Fiume which for good reason had not been included in the Pact of London, because it naturally belonged to the new Jugo-Slav state. Wilson consequently went to the public with his arguments, and the Italian delegation withdrew from the Conference.

With the Italians already turning their back on the League, the Japanese saw their chance to push for control of the Shantung Province in China. Wilson backed China's rights and lectured the nations on their duties toward each other. However, he did not want Japan to leave also and perhaps form an alliance with Russia and Germany; neither England nor America was willing to go to war with Japan over Shantung. Therefore it was agreed that Japan would control Shantung temporarily, and Wilson hoped that the League of Nations would later rectify the situation for China. Above all, Wilson struggled to save the League itself. The Italians never did get Fiume, but they did return to sign the final Treaty. By preventing an unjust decision, a war between the Jugo-Slavs and the Italians was made less likely. Wilson also compromised with the French on the Saar and Rhineland districts, and annexations were modified into temporary mandate agreements.

Germany had been suffering greatly; a food blockade by the Allies had been maintained against them for four months after the Armistice. Finally at the instigation of Herbert Hoover, President Wilson convinced the Allied leaders that the blockade must be lifted for humanitarian reasons. The Treaty agreed upon by the Allies and neutral nations was presented to the Germans on May 7. Their response on May 29 repeatedly complained of failures of the Treaty to adhere to the "Fourteen Points and subsequent addresses." They felt unnecessarily humiliated by the severe provisions the French had demanded. However, with the threat of Marshal Foch moving the French army in on them, the Germans decided to sign the Treaty. On June 28 the Treaty of Versailles was signed by Clemenceau, Lloyd George, Wilson, and other representatives of the nations.

Wilson was greeted by ten thousand people when he returned to New York. However, in the Senate there were strong isolationist sentiments against the Treaty. Presenting it to the Senate on July 10 President Wilson wondered forebodingly, "Dare we reject it and break the heart of the world?" A few "irreconcilables" were completely against the League. Many senators favored it, but ratification of a treaty required two-thirds of the Senate. A third group led by Senator Lodge demanded reservations, particularly to Article X of the League which read:

> The Members of the League undertake to respect and preserve as against external aggression the territorial integrity and existing political independence of all Members of the League. In case of any such aggression or in case of any threat or danger of such aggression the Council shall advise upon the means by which this obligation shall be fulfilled.

For Wilson this was the key article; it was the Monroe Doctrine applied to the world and protected by all. The President explained to the senators that this was a moral obligation but not necessarily a legal obligation. Senator Warren Harding asked what good it would do if it was only a moral obligation which a nation could ignore since it was not legally bound. Wilson pointed out that because it was not legally binding, the nation would have the right to exercise its moral judgment in each case. Lloyd George explained that the covenant did not necessarily imply "military action in support of the imperilled nation" but mainly economic pressure and sanctions against the aggressing nation. Former President Taft agreed that the chance of getting involved in a war was small because of the universal boycott which in most cases would be effective; only a world conspiracy would require the "union of overwhelming forces of the members of the League," and in that case "the earliest we get into the war, the better." Taft, a Republican, believed the United States could not be forced into a war against its will, and to think so was "a narrow and reactionary viewpoint."

Nevertheless opposition in the Senate was growing. Therefore President Wilson decided to take his case to the people with a busy speaking tour across the whole country. Young Americans had fought and died in France, and he would not give up the struggle for a world of peace without giving all he could. Wilson argued that the League of Nations was founded according to the American principles of self-government, open discussion and arbitration instead of war, a universal boycott of an offending nation, disarmament, rehabilitation of oppressed peoples, no annexations but trusteeships, abolition of forced labor especially of women and children, rejection of secret treaties, protection of dependent peoples, high standards of labor, the Red Cross, international regulation of drugs and alcohol, and prohibition of arms sales. He warned against violent revolutions such as had occurred in Russia rather than revolution by vote. The United States could be isolated no more, for "we have become a determining factor in the history of mankind" and in the development of civilization. He declared, "The peace of the world cannot be established without America." Seven and a half million men had been killed in the war; this was more than all the wars from 1793 to 1914. He spoke of the children who would have to die in a worse war if the League of Nations was not established. Wilson pushed himself to the limit, traveling 8,000 miles in twenty-two days and giving thirty-eight speeches. He had increasingly bad headaches which became constant until he finally collapsed in Pueblo, Colorado. The train took him straight back to Washington where he suffered a stroke, leaving the left side of his face and body paralyzed.

His wife coordinated his Presidential responsibilities. The push in the Senate for reservations to the Treaty was strong, but Wilson refused to give in because it would be repudiating what each nation had signed. If the United States demanded changes, then why could not the Germans also? Thus the President asked those who supported the Treaty to vote against ratification with the reservations, and consequently the Treaty was never ratified by the United States. Wilson hoped, perhaps, to be nominated again for President in 1920, but he was a broken man. The Republican Harding declared nebulously that he favored some sort of association of nations, and he was elected for "a return to normalcy." In Wilson's last public statement in 1923 he lamented, "I have seen fools resist Providence before." He still believed that his principles would eventually prevail. He died on February 3, 1924.

On January 16, 1920 President Wilson formally convoked the Council in accordance with the League provision for the summoning of the first Council and Assembly by the President of the United States. It was to be the last official participation by the United States in the entire history of the League of Nations. The League became a dead issue in American politics, and even Herbert Hoover and Franklin Roosevelt, who both had been early League supporters, could not get the United States involved during their Presidencies. The League, which the United States was expected to lead, lost its universal acceptance and credibility without the American power. Although virtually every other nation in the world joined the League, eventually several of the New World countries withdrew — Costa Rica and Brazil in the mid-twenties and Paraguay, Nicaragua, Honduras, Salvador, Chile, Venezuela, and Peru in the middle-to-late thirties.

Germany was admitted to the League in 1926 but withdrew in 1933. The debts and reparations were reduced and made more bearable for the German economy, and in the early thirties Hitler and the Nazi Party, using strong electioneering tactics, rose to power and began to re-arm. A Disarmament Conference was finally held in 1932-1933; but when Hitler and Germany withdrew after speaking sugar-coated words about peace, the disarmament process became futile. Japan's excursions in Manchuria during this period were tolerated, because the League did not refer to them as war. Japan also withdrew in 1933. Communist Russia was treated like an atheist pariah by League Members until fear of Germany and the diplomacy of Maxim Litvinov led to an invitation for the Soviet Union to join in 1934. The Saar district was returned to Germany when, with Nazi encouragement 90% of the people voted for German rule. Hitler completely repudiated the Versailles Treaty and sent troops to the Rhineland area, and by 1938 Germany could simply annex Austria without a complaint from the League. The most disastrous blow was when Italy under the Fascist leadership of Mussolini invaded and took over Ethiopia in 1936. The exiled Emperor of Ethiopia, Haile Selassie, made an eloquent appeal to the League for help against the Italians' mustard gas bombing of his weak nation. However, the most that the League had been able to do was to boycott Italy and Ethiopia; this hindered Italy little since the United States and others were still trading with them. Neither did the League do anything about the Nazi

146

bombing of Spain during its civil war.

Perhaps the League had helped to prevent small wars and through cooperation brought a little more collective consciousness into international affairs, but its failure became overwhelmingly obvious when the aggressions of Japan, Italy, and Germany brought on a second and greater world war that many had feared.

16
Franklin Roosevelt and the United Nations

"Truly, if the genius of mankind
that has invented the weapons of death
cannot discover the means of preserving peace,
civilization as we know it lives in an evil day."

Franklin Roosevelt

"Peace comes from the spirit and must be grounded in faith."

Franklin Roosevelt

"Freedom means the supremacy of human rights everywhere."

Franklin Roosevelt

"We the peoples of the United Nations determined
to save succeeding generations from the scourge of war,
which twice in our lifetime
has brought untold sorrow to mankind,
and to reaffirm faith in fundamental human rights,
in the dignity and worth of the human person,
in the equal rights of men and women
and of nations large and small,
and to establish conditions under which justice
and respect for the obligations arising from treaties
and other sources of international law can be maintained,
and to promote social progress
and better standards of life in larger freedom,
and for these ends to practice tolerance
and live together in peace with one another as good neighbors,
and to unite our strength
to maintain international peace and security,
and to ensure, by the acceptance of principles
and the institution of methods,
that armed force shall not be used,
save in the common interest,
and to employ international machinery for the promotion
of the economic and social advancement of all peoples,
have resolved to combine our efforts
to accomplish these aims."

Charter of the United Nations

*"Recognition of the inherent dignity
and of the equal and inalienable rights
of all members of the human family
is the foundation of freedom, justice, and peace in the world."*
Universal Declaration of Human Rights

As with Woodrow Wilson and the League of Nations, the primary initiator of the United Nations was an American President, Franklin Roosevelt. However, Roosevelt, the United States, and the world had learned from failures with the League. Roosevelt was not as closely identified with the UN as Wilson had been with the League, and he died shortly before the United Nations' founding conference and the termination of the Second World War.

Franklin Delano Roosevelt was born on January 30, 1882 at Hyde Park, New York. At Harvard young Franklin was not particularly studious, but he excelled in extra-curricular activities. He admired the progressive policies of President Theodore Roosevelt, who was his distant cousin, and he married TR's niece Eleanor Roosevelt. Eleanor was his lifelong partner in political work, and after his death she was a leading promoter of the United Nations. Franklin became a lawyer and was elected state senator in 1910 as a progressive Democrat. Roosevelt supported Woodrow Wilson for President, and he was appointed assistant secretary of the navy in 1913.

In July 1919 when the League of Nations was being debated, Roosevelt argued that the League was necessary for a successful peace settlement. He concluded hopefully, "If the League of Nations, with its future benefits to the world, is adopted, the future generations will look to us and call us blessed." In 1920 FDR was selected by the Democratic convention as their candidate for Vice President and running mate of James Cox. Roosevelt campaigned in favor of the League of Nations, saying that for the first time in history nations were being placed on the same basis as the relations between individuals so that an outlaw nation could not murder or maim "without being prevented from further misdeeds in the community of nations." He prophetically warned his country, "If you want the repetition of another war against civilization, then let us go back to the conditions of 1914. If you want the possibility of sending once more our troops and navies to foreign lands, then stay out of the League." He explained how Republican party leaders decided to sabotage the League in order to prevent a Republican defeat in the next Presidential election, even after President Wilson had met with Republican leaders and gotten the Monroe Doctrine incorporated into the League Covenant. Will Hays, Chairman of the Republican National Committee, secretly met with Senators Lodge, Borah, Brandegee and others and convinced them to follow a "deliberate and carefully planned campaign to throw over the treaty of peace and to discredit the President of the United States, in order to secure a victory for the Republican Party." Roosevelt continued, "The choice was made at that time. Partisan advantage was placed first, and the restoration of peace to civilization was thrown into the discard. As a result of that determination of more than one year ago, the restoration of peace still hangs in the balance." In the closing days of the campaign Roosevelt raised the moral question of the League versus the banking interests; he pointed out how educators, religious leaders, lawyers, organizations of mothers, and soldiers who fought in France favored the League because they were aware of the issues; but because the moneyed interests and eighty per cent of the newspapers were against the League, the ignorant majority would vote for the Republicans. The Republicans won the election.

Suddenly in August 1921 Franklin Roosevelt was struck with polio and was almost completely paralyzed. He regained the use of everything except his legs, but he remained physically crippled in the legs for the rest of his life. However, he refused to retire, as his mother suggested, and he stayed active in politics with Eleanor's help. In 1924 he proposed a new international organization to replace the League, and at the Democratic convention he nominated his fellow New Yorker, Governor Al Smith, for President. Smith urged him to run for governor in 1928, and Roosevelt was elected and re-elected in 1930.

In 1932 Roosevelt wrestled the Presidential nomination away from Smith and won a big victory over Hoover during the depth of the Depression. As President, Roosevelt took immediate action to meet the crisis with his various New Deal programs of recovery for a blighted economy. He was overwhelmingly re-elected in 1936, but had difficulty with the Supreme Court and a recession in 1937. Roosevelt had brought a creative and dynamic activity to government to deal with massive economic problems based on his real concern for the poor, the unemployed, and the destitute. His programs attempted to establish economic and social security for all Americans.

His first major foreign policy speech was on Woodrow Wilson's birthday at the end of 1933. He clearly defined United States policy as being opposed to armed intervention. In an unusual statement for a politician, he admitted, "The blame for the danger to world peace lies not in the world population but in the political leaders." He recalled how the masses of people had enthusiastically responded to Wilson's gallant appeal and how political profit, personal prestige, and national aggrandizement had handicapped the League's inception. Roosevelt believed "that the old policies, alliances, combinations and balances of power have proved themselves inadequate for the preservation of world peace. The League of Nations, encouraging as it does the extension of nonaggression pacts, of reduction of armament agreements, is a prop in the world peace structure." Perhaps the same is true of the United Nations today, and the same challenge that Wilson and Roosevelt faced we still face today, which is, as FDR stated, "whether people themselves could not some day prevent governments from making war." Although it was politically impossible for the American President to get the United States involved in the League, Roosevelt did encourage cooperation with the non-political and humanitarian work of League agencies. In 1940 he wrote, "However governments may divide, human problems are common the world over and we shall never realize peace until these common interests take precedence as the major work of civilization."

In a speech on October 5, 1937 Roosevelt spoke out against the worsening world situation caused by violations of treaties and undeclared acts of war that killed innocent civilians. He warned that America would not be safe from the contagion of war. He asserted that peace-loving nations must attempt to uphold laws and treaties, because in international anarchy there is no escape through isolation. "Those who cherish their freedom and recognize and respect the equal right of their neighbors to be free and live in peace, must work together for the triumph of law and moral principles in order that peace, justice and confidence may prevail in the world." He pointed out how much of the world's economy was being spent on armaments. The President believed that America must actively engage in the search for peace, and he suggested a quarantine against the epidemic of aggressor nations. Thus the policy of the United States was no loner isolation, and shortly a League committee declared that Japan was the aggressor against China.

A year later Roosevelt pleaded with Hitler to settle the differences between Germany and Czechoslovakia by peaceful means, but Hitler marched his troops into that country. In April 1939 Roosevelt again appealed to Hitler and Mussolini to prevent the disaster of war. Speaking from strength and human friendship he asked these dictators not to invade thirty independent nations he named, and he proposed negotiations to reduce the crushing economic burdens of armaments and to open international trade. Finally one week before the war broke out, FDR sent an appeal to Hitler, King Victor Emmanuel of Italy, and President Moscicki of Poland, but only the Polish leader was interested in averting war.

When war was declared, President Roosevelt sent messages to Great Britain, France, Italy, Germany, and Poland requesting that they not bomb civilians. In a fireside chat to the nation on September 3, 1939 he declared that the policy of the United States was neutrality, but he did not expect people to be neutral in their minds and consciences. He hoped that America would be able to stay out of the war.

After winning an unprecedented third term as President, at the end of 1940 Roosevelt declared that America must become "the great arsenal democracy" to economically aid the Allies against the Fascists' warfare. Then he gave his famous "4 freedoms" speech in January 1941. America had been founded on the first two freedoms of religion and speech. Roosevelt's response to the

Depression and World War II was to call for freedom from want and freedom from fear. Not only did he believe that all Americans deserved these rights, but also everyone in the world. Roosevelt said that freedom from want "means economic understandings which will secure to every nation a healthy peacetime life for its inhabitants — everywhere in the world," and freedom from fear "means a world-wide reduction of armaments to such a point and in such a thorough fashion that no nation will be in a position to commit an act of physical aggression against any neighbor — anywhere in the world."

In August 1941 Roosevelt and Winston Churchill, the Prime Minister for the United Kingdom, agreed on the Atlantic Charter which declared their nations' principles and intentions in regard to the circumstances of the war. First, they sought no territorial aggrandizement. Second, they wanted no territorial changes that would not be in "accord with the freely expressed wishes of the peoples concerned." Third, they respected the right of all peoples to self-government. Fourth, they supported states' equal access to trade and the raw materials of the world. Fifth, they wished to promote economic cooperation, "improved labor standards, economic advancement, and social security." Sixth, after destroying the Nazi tyranny they hoped to establish a peace that would be secure to all nations and peoples in freedom from fear and want. Seventh, this peace would include freedom of the seas. Eighth and last, they declared, "All of the nations of the world, for realistic as well as spiritual reasons, must come to the abandonment of the use of force. Since no future peace can be maintained if land, sea, or air armaments continue to be employed by nations which threaten, or may threaten, aggression outside of their frontiers, they believe, pending the establishment of a wider and permanent system of general security, that the disarmament of such nations is essential. They will likewise aid and encourage all other practicable measures which will lighten for peaceloving peoples the crushing burden of armaments." The "they" refers to the two signers, Franklin D. Roosevelt and Winston S. Churchill.

With the surprise attack on the United States by the Japanese on December 7, 1941 America was drawn fully into the war.

When Churchill and the Soviet Ambassador Litvinov met with Roosevelt in Washington to confirm the new alliance against the Axis powers, FDR suggested the name "United Nations." On January 1, 1942 these representatives along with Soong of China signed the Declaration of the United Nations "to defend life, liberty, independence, and religious freedom, and to preserve human rights and justice in their own lands as well as in other lands." The pact was later signed by the other twenty-two nations named in the declaration. More than three years later when the name of the new international organization was being discussed in San Francisco, the name "United Nations" was selected as a tribute to Roosevelt.

Roosevelt conceived the organization as world-wide in scope, although important decisions would be made by the United States, Great Britain, Russia, and China, who would have the responsibility of policing the world. This is what he told the British Foreign Minister Anthony Eden and Churchill in March 1943. On November 1, Secretary of State Cordell Hull, Eden, Soviet Foreign Minister Molotov, and the Chinese Ambassador to Moscow signed the Moscow Declaration in which the four powers agreed to maintain international peace after the war, and they stated, "That they recognize the necessity of establishing at the earliest practicable date a general international organization, based on the principle of the sovereign equality of all peace-loving states, and open to membership by all such states, large and small, for the maintenance of international peace and security." This statement was incorporated into the Connally Resolution and was passed by the United States Senate on November 6, 1943. Already Congress was on record in favor of a world organization. On November 9, representatives of forty-four nations met at the White House and established the United Nations Relief and Rehabilitation Administration (UNRRA).

At the end of November 1943 Roosevelt met with Churchill and Stalin at Tehran, and FDR began to share his outline of the organization for the preservation of world peace. The Assembly would include all members of the United Nations and would be world-wide in scope; they would discuss world problems and recommend solutions. The Executive Committee would be composed of the U.S.S.R., the U.S., the U.K., and China along with representatives of two European nations, one South American, one Middle Eastern, one Far Eastern, and one British Dominion. They would deal with all nonmilitary questions such as economy, food, health, etc., but both Stalin and Roosevelt were reluctant to give them any binding power. The third group would be "The Four Policemen" (U.S.S.R., U.S., U.K., and China). They would have the power to use force against any threat to the peace. Both Stalin and Churchill suggested regional committees, but Roosevelt did not expect the forces of China or the U.S. to be needed in Europe. Apparently the possibility of one of the Four Policemen being an aggressor was not discussed. The conference concluded amicably with Roosevelt saying how nations with different customs and philosophies could blend in harmony like the colors of a rainbow for the common good.

In his annual message to Congress in January 1944 Roosevelt proposed an "economic Bill of Rights." He said that security means not only safety from attacks by aggressors but also "economic security, social security, moral security — in a family of nations." He felt that these rights should include earning enough from a job for food, clothing, and recreation, buying and selling products, a decent home, medical care, and education.

In August 1944 representatives of the Big Four met at the Dumbarton Oaks Conference in Washington. The Russians insisted that the Chinese be excluded until the major decisions were made by the other three powers. The tentative American plan had two broad purposes for the international organization: to preserve peace and security, and to promote international cooperation on economic and social problems. The plan now had five functional divisions; in addition to a General Assembly and Executive Council, there would be an International Court, a Secretariat, and subsidiary agencies. Security questions were to be solely vested in the Executive Council which now would include France as a fifth permanent member and six rotating members. Any one of the five permanent members would be able to block an action in regard to disputes, settlements, sanctions, and uses of force. There was still a question whether one of the five powers could use this veto if that nation was itself involved in the dispute.

The Americans went along with the British in proposing that a veto not be allowed by a power who was a party to a dispute. The Soviet representative Gromyko responded to this by requesting that all sixteen Soviet republics be included as charter members of the UN. Roosevelt felt that "this might ruin the chance of getting an international organization accepted publicly in this country." With the abeyance of these two questions, the American tentative proposals were generally accepted. A compromise on the veto issue was suggested on September 13 and was later adopted in the UN Charter. A permanent member could veto any use of force even if it was a party to a dispute, but it could not veto a decision which came under "Pacific Settlement of Disputes" if it was a party to the dispute.

Roosevelt was elected to a fourth term as President, and in his Inaugural Address on January 20, 1945 he spoke of the lessons the United States had learned from the war — "that we cannot live alone, at peace; that our own well-being is dependent on the well-being of other nations — far away . . . We have learned to be citizens of the world, members of the human community. We have learned the simple truth, Emerson said, that 'the only way to have a friend is to be one.' We can gain no lasting peace if we approach it with suspicion and mistrust — and with fear."

Roosevelt met again with Churchill and Stalin at Yalta in February 1945. Stalin agreed to the veto solution but insisted on at least two extra votes for the Ukraine and Byelorussia in the General Assembly. Since it would not affect the Executive Council and as a gesture of goodwill toward the Russians who had had twenty million killed fighting the Nazis, Roosevelt accepted this proposal, if the UN conference they scheduled to begin in San Francisco on April 25 would also accept the two additional Russian republics after discussion and a free vote. Roosevelt considered the Crimean Conference more successful than the peace efforts made a quarter of a century earlier. He believed that a universal organization of all peace-loving nations should mark the end of methods such as unilateral action, exclusive alliances, spheres of influence, and balances of power which had failed for centuries. On March 1 he reported to the Congress about the Crimean Conference saying how the Senate was being advised of the new international security organization and declaring, "World peace is not a party question." World peace cannot depend upon the work of one man, one party, or one nation, or even the large nations or the small nations. "It must be a peace which rests on the cooperative effort of the whole world." In a press conference on April 5, Roosevelt expressed the view that for the Soviet Union to have three votes in the General Assembly was not that significant because it was only an investigative body that really would not decide important issues.

Franklin Roosevelt died on April 12, 1945. On that day he wrote a speech to be given in honor of Thomas Jefferson's birthday on April 13. He looked past the conquest of the malignant Nazi state toward the conquest of the root causes — doubts, fears, ignorance, and greed. He asked us to face the fact that "if civilization is to survive, we must cultivate the science of human relationships — the ability of all peoples, of all kinds, to live together and work together in the same world, at peace . . . The work, my friends, is peace, more than an end of this war — an end to the beginning of all wars, yes, an end, forever, to this impractical, unrealistic settlement of the differences between governments by the mass killing of peoples." In his last words he appealed to people to dedicate themselves to peace and act with faith. "The only limit to our realization of tomorrow will be our doubts of today. Let us move forward with strong and active faith."

Delegates of fifty nations met in San Francisco on April 25 for the United Nations Conference on International Organization. Using the Dumbarton Oaks proposals as a basis they worked in committees and plenary sessions to draw up the 111-article Charter which was adopted unanimously on June 25, 1945. The Charter became effective the following October 24 after China, France, the USSR, the United Kingdom, the United States, and a majority of the signing nations had ratified the document.

The Charter defines the purposes of the United Nations as the maintenance of peace and security in accordance with justice and international law, friendly relations among nations based on equal rights and self-determination of peoples, and international cooperation on solving economic, social, cultural, and humanitarian problems with respect for human rights. All members agree to "settle their international disputes by peaceful means" and to "refrain from the threat or use of force against the territorial integrity or political independence of any state."

Article 26 begins, "In order to promote the establishment and maintenance of international peace and security with the least diversion for armaments of the world's human and economic resources," and it sets up a committee to work to establish "a system for the regulation of armaments." Chapter VI entitled "Pacific Settlement of Disputes" begins with Article 33: "The parties to any dispute, the continuance of which is likely to endanger the maintenance of international peace and security, shall, first of all, seek a solution by negotiation, enquiry, mediation, conciliation, arbitration, judicial settlement, resort to regional agencies or arrangements, or other peaceful means of their own choice." The Security Council may request parties to use such means, may investigate disputes, and may make recommendations. Chapter VII discusses actions which may be taken to maintain or restore international peace when there are threats to the peace, breaches of the peace, and acts of aggression. The Security Council may decide to use force or economic sanctions and call upon member nations to make available armed forces, assistance, and facilities. Chapter VIII states that regional arrangements for maintaining peace are not precluded by the Charter.

When Harry Truman became President and the atomic bomb was developed, the relations of the United States toward Russia and the UN began to change into the Cold War. Lend-Lease aid to Russia was ended on May 12, 1945, while Great Britain was granted a low-interest loan. Soviet fears of an international bloc against them were also fed by America's support for regional blocs' use of collective self-defense, which reversed the U.S. position at Dumbarton Oaks. Truman also decided to use the atomic bomb as a bargaining factor in dealing with the Russians, and he attempted to negate Roosevelt's abandonment of control over Eastern Europe. In October 1945 Truman saw the UN as the only alternative to "a bitter armament race with the Russians."

By 1947 the failure of the Security Council to organize the forces necessary for the collective security framework in which disarmament could have been established allowed the Cold War arms race to dominate the international scene. Meanwhile the permanent members of the Security Council were getting around their partial ban of the veto if they were a party to a dispute simply by not calling it a "dispute."

The Cold War became hot in Korea in 1950. The armies of the US and USSR had occupied Korea in 1945 to accept the surrender of Japanese troops on each side of the 38th parallel. A UN Commission observed elections in South Korea in 1948 but was refused access to North Korea. In June 1950 North Korean forces invaded the Republic of Korea. Since the USSR had stopped attending the Security Council in protest over the representation of China, the Council was able to recommend that members send armed forces to restore security to South Korea. After the additional intervention of the People's Republic of China and much fighting, an armistice finally stopped hostilities in July 1953.

In November 1950 the western powers also took advantage of Russia's absence from the Security Council to pass the "Uniting for Peace" resolution, which enables the General Assembly to recommend collective measures for maintaining peace if the Security Council does not fulfill its peacekeeping responsibility because of lack of unanimity among its permanent members. The USSR soon returned to the Security Council so that it could make effective use of its veto.

Even if the veto could be circumvented, the capabilities of nuclear weapons have made action against an offending super-power too risky, as the reluctance to intervene in Hungary in 1956 and Czechoslovakia in 1968 has made clear. The deterrence of nuclear weapons has essentially replaced the collective system of deterrence if the nuclear powers are involved. Since Korea, the Cold War has prevented the use of the large powers' forces as UN police, which was the original intention, because of mutual fear. Instead the forces of small countries have been employed to stop small wars and hostilities in such places as Palestine, Pakistan-

India, Indonesia, Congo, Cypress, Israel and the Sinai, Syria, and Lebanon. The UN has supported decolonization, and economic sanctions were imposed on Rhodesia because of its flagrant violations of human rights.

The United Nations has difficulty keeping states in line against their will, but the veto has at least kept the super-powers talking together in the Security Council, even though they may not be able to agree. The General Assembly is a great public forum for the debate of international issues, and the developments of the economic and social functions have made progress in dealing with many of the root causes of war.

The cornerstone of this powerful cathedral for the voices of public opinion has been the Universal Declaration of Human Rights, which was adopted unanimously by the General Assembly on December 10, 1948. Eleanor Roosevelt, who was the chairman (chairperson) of the Commission on Human Rights which drew up the document, explained why eight members abstained from the unanimous vote. The Soviets and their satellites asserted that the Declaration failed to recognize more than the eighteenth century rights and did not adequately emphasize the new economic and social rights of the twentieth century; South Africa characteristically felt the opposite — that the rights granted were too modern; and Saudi Arabia objected to an individual's "right to change his religion or belief."

Nevertheless the Universal Declaration of Human Rights elucidates an ideal modern standard of freedoms, rights, and responsibilities for all people and nations. The United Nations promotes through education respect for these rights and freedoms. Among the many rights included in the thirty articles are the following: human equality and brotherhood; non-discrimination by race, color, sex, language, religion, politics, nationality, property, birth, or social status; life, liberty, and security; no slavery; no torture or cruel punishment; equality before the law; recourse to law for violations; no arbitrary arrest; fair trial against criminal charges with presumption of innocence until proof of guilt, and no retroactive penal laws; privacy and protection of the law; freedom of movement within one's state and to leave and return to one's country; nationality and the right to change it; marriage by free choice and family; ownership of property; freedom of thought, conscience, and religion; freedom of expression including media; freedom of assembly and association; participation in government, free elections, and equal access to public services. The economic, social, and cultural rights include the following: choice of employment under good conditions and protection against unemployment; equal pay for equal work and fair remuneration; trade unions; rest, leisure, limited working hours, and paid holidays; health and medical care with special care for all mothers and children; free elementary education and equal access to technical and professional education; education shall promote human rights and universal friendship among all people; parents may choose their children's education; participation in cultural life, arts, and the benefits of science; protection of authorship in science, literature, and art; social and international order that realizes these rights; one's duties to the community include subjection to laws which protect others' rights.

On December 16, 1966 the General Assembly adopted many of these rights to be ratified into law by willing nations in the International Covenant on Economic, Social and Cultural Rights and the International Covenant on Civil and Political Rights, both of which entered into force in those countries that ratified them in January 1976. The Charter of Economic Rights and Duties of States which granted sovereignty over wealth and natural resources was adopted by the General Assembly on December 12, 1974.

The United Nations is far from perfect and complete as a world organization, but it has enabled humanity to take many important steps on the path of social evolution. The peacekeeping problems of the arms race and nuclear weaponry and the effective enforcement of international law will be discussed further in Chapter 21, which covers world law and disarmament.

161

17

Einstein and Schweitzer on Peace in the Atomic Age

*"Every thoughtful, well-meaning and conscientious human being
should assume, in time of peace,
the solemn and unconditional obligation
not to participate in any war, for any reason,
or to lend support of any kind, whether direct or indirect."*
Albert Einstein

*"The unleashed power of the atom has changed everything
save our modes of thinking,
and thus we drift toward unparalleled catastrophe."*
Albert Einstein

*"Mankind's desire for peace can be realized
only by the creation of a world government."*
Albert Einstein

*"The highest insight man can attain is the yearning for peace,
for the union of his will with an infinite will,
his human will with God's will."*
Albert Schweitzer

"The peace of God is pulsating power, not quietude."
Albert Schweitzer

*"The laying down of the commandment not to kill
and not to damage is one of the greatest events
in the spiritual history of mankind."*
Albert Schweitzer

*"Only a humanity which is striving after ethical ends
can in full measure share in the blessings
brought by material progress
and become master of the dangers which accompany it."*
Albert Schweitzer

"The renunciation of nuclear weapons is vital to peace."
Albert Schweitzer

Albert Einstein, the renowned scientist whose theories of relativity led to the development of atomic energy and weapons, was a dedicated pacifist and advocate of world government. He was born March 14, 1879 in Ulm, Germany. He grew up in Munich where he attended strict schools in which he performed poorly. His mother insisted he take violin lessons, and his uncles introduced him to mathematics and science. At the age of 5 he wondered why a compass always pointed north, and at 12 he began a quest to understand the mystery of the "huge world." He continued to have difficulty in school until he moved to Switzerland where in 1900 he graduated in physics from the reputable Polytechnic Academy in Zurich. He gained Swiss citizenship and got a job in the patent office in Bern examining inventions.

In 1905 Einstein began to publish important papers in theoretical physics, particularly on the special theory of relativity, which synthesized the law of the conservation of the mass with the law of the conservation of energy into an equivalence in terms of the speed of light squared: $E = mc^2$. The three dimensional coordinates of space and the one of time were also joined into the four dimensional continuum of space-time. Einstein gained some recognition from eminent physicists and began teaching at universities in Switzerland and Germany. He moved his family to Berlin in April 1914 to accept a position with the Prussian Academy. His wife and two sons were vacationing in Switzerland when the war broke out, and the enforced separation foreshadowed a later divorce. Einstein hated the war and criticized German militarism, as we shall see, but he devoted himself to his scientific work. He published "The Foundation of the General Theory of Relativity" in 1916. Using the space-time continuum concept he postulated that gravity is not a force as much as a field shaped by bodies of mass. His theory was proved correct when he accurately predicted that even light from stars would bend when passing near the sun; this was measured and verified by Arthur Eddington during a total eclipse in 1919. Einstein was now internationally acclaimed as perhaps the greatest scientist of the twentieth century. In 1921 he was awarded the Nobel Prize for Physics. Einstein spent the rest of his scientific career working on his unified field theory, attempting to find the mathematical relationship between the electromagnetic field and the gravitational field. However, quantum theory and the uncertainty principle thwarted his efforts to find a formula which could predict subatomic events. Einstein clung to his belief that the universe is comprehensible, saying that God does not play dice with the world.

As a world-famous celebrity Einstein's statements on peace were given considerable publicity. When the first World War began, Einstein and two others signed a statement by Georg Friedrich Nicholai challenging the "Manifesto to Europeans," which was a blatant promotion of German militarism that had been signed by ninety-three prominent Germans. Nicolai's statement warned that every nation in the war would pay a heavy price, and he suggested a League of Europeans to achieve unity. During the war Einstein was a founder and supporter of the New Fatherland League which sought to establish after the war a supranational organization to prevent future wars. He gleefully smuggled pacifist literature to his friend Nicholai in prison. In 1915 he signed a declaration by this League criticizing annexationist policies of the Chancellor. In a letter to the French pacifist writer, Romain Rolland, Einstein compared the "insanity of nationalism" to the religious fanaticism of three centuries earlier which had caused so many useless wars. In 1917 he wrote again to Rolland suggesting a "military arbitration pact among America, Britain, France and Russia" which any democratic nation could join. Although Einstein was not religious in the traditional sense, he was proud of being a Jew. Within the war atmosphere that swept up so many around him, he wrote to an academic, "I prefer to string along with my compatriot, Jesus Christ, whose doctrines you and your kind consider to be obsolete. Suffering is indeed more acceptable to me than resort to violence." Late in 1918 when Germany was undergoing revolution, Einstein gave a speech at the Reichstag suggesting to the revolutionary committees, "Our common goal is democracy, the rule of the people," but warning them, "Do not be lured by feelings of vengeance to the fateful view that violence must be fought with violence, that a dictatorship of the

164

proletariat is temporarily needed in order to hammer the concept of freedom into the heads of our fellow countrymen. Force breeds only bitterness, hatred and reaction."

After the war Einstein favored the publication of the war crimes committed by the German High Command in Belgium and France to communicate to Germans how the others felt in order to "prevent the emergence of a spirit of vengefulness." In 1922 he made a trip to Paris to discuss with political figures methods of preventing wars, and returning to Germany he spoke again in the Reichstag at a meeting of the German Peace Federation calling for goodwill between peoples of different languages and cultures. In a German pacifist publication Einstein explained how war blocks international cooperation and culture by destroying intellectual freedom, chaining the energies of the young to the engines of destruction, and causing economic depression.

Einstein supported the League of Nations, but he resigned from the League Committee on Intellectual Cooperation in 1923 when France did not agree to arbitration concerning Germany's war-reparations payment. He felt that the League was merely a tool of the dominant nations. In 1924 he was re-elected to that Committee and decided to "let bygones be bygones" and accept the position, hoping that the League would "live up to its great mission of creating a world of peace."

In 1928 Einstein began recommending that individuals refuse military service and any participation in war activities. During this period Einstein's pacifism was absolute, and he believed that any killing of a human being, even during war, is murder. He saw how science and technology were changing warfare, and he believed that international conventions to limit the applications of science did not solve the real problem, which was how to end war by establishing international justice. In pleading for disarmament, Einstein felt that its risks and sacrifices were less than the risks and sacrifices of war. People ought to refuse to kill other innocent people. However, he saw that Europe was systematically preparing for war, and he predicted, "An impotent League of Nations will not be able to command even moral authority in the hour of nationalist madness." The production of armaments, for Einstein, was damaging not only economically but also spiritually. In 1930 he signed a manifesto for world disarmament sponsored by the Women's International League for Peace and Freedom. The same year Einstein warned the Zionist movement that he would not continue to support them unless they made peace with the Arabs. On December 14, 1930 Einstein made his famous statement in New York that if two per cent of those called for military service were to refuse to fight and were to urge peaceful means of settling international conflicts, then governments would become powerless since they could not imprison that many people. He struggled against compulsory military service and urged international protection of conscientious objectors. He concluded that peace, freedom for individuals and security for societies depended on disarmament; otherwise, "slavery of the individual and the annihilation of civilization threaten us."

As part of his work for intellectual cooperation Einstein wrote an open letter to Sigmund Freud in 1932 asking him to discuss the causes and cures of war. In his letter Einstein suggested that an international legislative and judicial body was needed to solve conflicts and maintain security. In his carefully reasoned response Freud came to the same conclusion that Einstein had intuitively grasped. Later that year Einstein supported the French Premier Herriot's proposal for "a police force which would be subject to the authority of international organs." Early in 1933 Einstein warned that powerful industrial interests which produce arms were trying to sabotage efforts to settle international disputes peacefully.

When Hitler and the Nazi Party came to power in 1933 Einstein left Germany for good and settled at Princeton, where he joined the Institute for Advanced Study. He saw that Germany was "secretly arming at a great pace," and noticing "the desire for revenge among the educated," he predicted "the sacrifice of a terrifying number of human lives and untold destruction." Being realistic about this danger he ceased to be an absolute pacifist; although he still recommended a supranational organization of force, in its absence he felt that the democracies ought to prepare to defend themselves. He was criticized by some pacifists, but

Einstein felt that it would be foolish to close one's eyes to the Nazi menace. He tried to communicate the dreadfulness of Fascism and the Nazis' fanatical drive toward war. He encouraged the United States to join the League of Nations and to make it an effective instrument of international security. By 1935 he estimated that war would come in two or three years. He reiterated the need for world government: "First, create the idea of supersovereignty: men must be taught to think in world terms; every country will have to surrender a portion of its sovereignty through international cooperation." In 1937 he declared that true pacifism works for international law, while neutrality and isolation practiced by a great power contribute to international anarchy and consequently to war.

Einstein's famous formula $E = mc^2$ indicates that a very small amount of matter may be converted into a tremendous amount of energy. In July 1939 Leo Szilard told Einstein about the work under way which showed that through nuclear fission a chain reaction might be started. This was a shock to Einstein. Four and a half years earlier he had discounted the likelihood of releasing energy from a molecule, saying, "It is something like shooting birds in the dark in a country where there are only a few birds." Now he immediately realized the danger if Germany were to get uranium from the Belgian Congo, and he agreed to contact the Belgium government through his friend, Queen Elizabeth. Alexander Sachs, one of President Roosevelt's unofficial advisors, suggested to Einstein that he address a letter directly to the President. On August 2, 1939 Einstein wrote to President Roosevelt explaining how nuclear chain reactions in a large mass of uranium could generate large amounts of power and radium-like elements. In fact, in the immediate future, a powerful enough bomb could be built to destroy an entire port. He pointed out that the best uranium is found in Canada, the former Czechoslovakia, and especially the Belgian Congo, and he had heard that Germany had stopped the sale of uranium from the Czechoslovakian mines. He added, "The son of the German Under-Secretary of State, von Weiszäcker, is attached to the Kaiser Wilhelm Institut in Berlin, where some of the American work on uranium is now being repeated." The letter, with a

167

memorandum by Szilard, actually was not delivered to the President by Sachs until October 11. President Roosevelt immediately appointed an Advisory Committee on Uranium. Later Einstein considered the writing of this letter the one great mistake of his life; at the time he felt justified because of the danger that the Germans would make atom bombs. This was the extent of Einstein's role in nuclear energy; he did not know an atomic bomb had been developed by the United States until he heard of the Hiroshima blast.

For the rest of his life Einstein emphasized the need for a supranational organization with the authority and power to maintain international security. With the unleashing of the atomic bomb in 1945 his pleas became even more fervent. As a knowledgeable scientist he felt that it was his responsibility to inform the public of the enormity of the danger. The United Nations was a step in the right direction, but from the beginning Einstein believed that it was "a tragic illusion unless we are ready to take the further steps necessary to organize peace." There must be effective world law with a Federal Constitution and a permanent world court to restrain the executive branch of the world government from going beyond peace-keeping. National military power must be abandoned in favor of the supranational authority. Otherwise war preparations inevitably lead to war, and in the atomic age there is the danger of pre-emptive war and the possibility of total annihilation. Einstein supported efforts to strengthen the United Nations and give it the powers it needs. Survival, he felt, must be the first priority, and survival depends on world government. There is no defense against nuclear weapons. Einstein evaluated every nation's foreign policy by one criterion: "Does it lead us to a world of law and order or does it lead us back toward anarchy and death?" He said, "We need a great chain reaction of awareness and communication."

Einstein criticized as political exploitation the policy of stockpiling atomic bombs without promising not to initiate their use. In 1947 only the United States had atomic weapons; however, the cold war had already begun, and the Soviet Union was developing them also. Both sides refused to consider supranational control, and Einstein lamented that the victors of the second world war had degraded themselves to the low ethics of their enemy and remained at that level after the war. In 1948 Einstein predicted that the arms race would increase tension between the United States and the Soviet Union, undermine the democratic spirit in America, impose heavy and unnecessary economic burdens due to the unproductive work, and generate that militaristic spirit which Toynbee said is fatal to civilizations. For Einstein, the problem of peace and security was far more important than the conflict between socialism and capitalism.

Einstein worked with the Emergency Committee of Atomic Scientists to educate people about the dangers of atomic war and the necessity of effective world government. By 1949 the Soviet Union had atomic weapons, and the United States had begun working on the hydrogen bomb. Einstein's prophecy that the cold war would threaten democratic principles in the United States came to pass with the operations of the House Un-American Activities Committee (HUAC). He recommended that intellectuals use Gandhi's method of non-cooperation by refusing to testify. Einstein believed that Gandhi held the most enlightened political views and that his method of non-violent revolution is the only way of bringing peace to the world on a supranational basis. With this method the small countries together could become a decisive factor in the world. Nevertheless he felt that a responsible statesman would not use Gandhi's methods unilaterally until there had been a period of transition.

In the last week of his life Einstein collaborated with Bertrand Russell on a manifesto concluding with a resolution to be presented to a world convention of scientists which read:

> In view of the fact that in any future world war nuclear weapons will certainly be employed, and that such weapons threaten the continued existence of mankind, we urge the governments of the world to realize, and to acknowledge publicly, that their purposes cannot be furthered by a world war, and we urge them, consequently, to find peaceful means for the settlement of all matters of dispute between them.

When Einstein died on April 18, 1955 he left a piece of writing ending in an unfinished sentence. There were his last words:

In essence, the conflict that exists today is no more than an old-style struggle for power, once again presented to mankind in semireligious trappings. The difference is that, this time, the development of atomic power has imbued the struggle with a ghostly character; for both parties know and admit that, should the quarrel deteriorate into actual war, mankind is doomed. Despite this knowledge, statesmen in responsible positions on both sides continue to employ the well-known technique of seeking to intimidate and demoralize the opponent by marshaling superior military strength. They do so even though such a policy entails the risk of war and doom. Not one statesman in a position of responsibility has dared to pursue the only course that holds out any promise of peace, the course of supranational security, since for a statesman to follow such a course would be tantamount to political suicide. Political passions, once they have been fanned into flame, exact their victims . . .

After Einstein's death Albert Schweitzer wrote to Einstein's niece that he and the great physicist understood each other and that they had the same ideals. Schweitzer was born four years before Einstein on January 14, 1875 in Alsace, which at that time was part of Germany but now is part of France. His father was a Lutheran pastor, and Albert studied and gained doctorate degrees in both philosophy and theology. He was an accomplished organist; he wrote a comprehensive book on Bach and later edited Bach's complete works. His theological books combined his deep religious convictions with a scholarly search for historical truth. Beyond the historical considerations he found the essence of Jesus' teachings to be love and "the preparation of the heart for the Kingdom." He concludes *Quest of the Historical Jesus* with Jesus' call for people to follow Him. "He commands. And to those who obey, be they wise or simple, He will reveal Himself through all that they are privileged to experience in His fellowship of peace and activity, of struggle and suffering, till they come to know, as an inexpressible secret, Who He is."

At the age of thirty Schweitzer decided to become a physician so that he could dedicate himself to practical missionary work. He resigned from his university teaching position and attended medical school full-time. His theological views were considered controversial by the mission officials. However, by making personal contacts with each of them to assure them he was going as a doctor rather than a preacher, he was granted the opportunity to serve in French Equatorial Africa at Lambaréné. His wife trained as a nurse, and by 1913 they were prepared. His farewell sermon was on "The Peace of God," which comes when our will is absorbed in the infinite. This, he said, must be our active search, and those who experience God's peace can face any eventuality. Sensing a coming war he had their money converted into coins before they left.

Schweitzer quickly gained the trust of the Africans in his medical practice; but when the world war began, Schweitzer, as a German, became a prisoner of the French authorities. The native Africans could not understand such a terrible war. One old man, hearing that as many as ten people had died, wondered why they did not negotiate a settlement since such great losses could not be paid back. According to their tribal customs they reimbursed the opposite tribe for those they killed. Also they felt that the Europeans must kill out of cruelty if they have no desire to eat the dead. Schweitzer was a prisoner for three years, although much of the time he was allowed to continue his work at the hospital. He began working on his *Philosophy of Civilization,* and while paddling down the Ogowe River in the midst of a herd of hippopotami the concept "reverence for life" suddenly occurred to him. He was taken to France, and while imprisoned at Saint-Remy he realized that he was in a room that Van Gogh had painted.

At the end of the war Schweitzer's first sermon at St. Nicholai's Church in Strasbourg was again on peace and also on the future of mankind. He repeated that we must place our will in God's infinite will and look for that, not only in individual affairs but also in the concerns of nations and mankind. The will of God is a spiritual intention toward perfection, and people as a whole must be united by spiritual goals. In another sermon on December 1, 1918 he said, "Those millions who were made to kill, forced to do it in self-defense or under military orders, must impress the horror of what they had to endure on all future generations so that none will ever expose itself to such fate again. Reverence for human suffering and human life, for the smallest and most insignificant, must be the inviolable law to rule the world from now on."

The huge waste of life during the war terribly grieved Schweitzer, and he was deeply depressed for several years. The war, he believed, was proof that religion was not a real force in the spiritual life of the age. Looking back on his first visit to Africa, he considered his work there not benevolence but rather atonement for a tiny part of the guilt the white race bears for all it has done to the colored races. Schweitzer hailed the League of Nations but was afraid that it would fail; he remained apolitical.

In *The Decay and the Restoration of Civilization* Schweitzer examines the problems of civilization and their solution through ethics. Nationalism has helped to bring about the decay of civilization because of the spirit of barbarism. Even the economic difficulties can be solved only "by an inner change of character." Revolutionary change is needed without revolutionary action. When the collective body dominates the individual's spiritual and moral worthiness, the constriction causes deterioration. The individuals must rise to a higher conception of their capabilities and produce new spiritual-ethical ideas. A new public opinion must be created to counteract the press which is under the influence of political and financial forces. This requires independent and strong personalities who are free of the prevalent conditions. Nationalistic patriotism must be replaced by the noble "patriotism which aims at ends that are worthy of the whole of mankind." This idealism encourages people to focus on the values of civilization even amid the increasing absorption in material concerns.

Nothing less than a reconstruction of the world-view can bring about such changes. The lack of a positive and life-affirming world-view is pathological to societies as well as individuals, since there is no true self-direction. Schweitzer declares, "From the ethical comes ability to develop the purposive state of mind necessary to produce action on the world and society and to cause the co-operation of all our achievements to secure the spiritual and moral perfection of the individual which is the final end of civilization."

The second book in his Philosophy of Civilization, *Civilization and Ethics,* reviews the history of ethics and its relation to civilization. For Schweitzer, ethics is the key to peace. "All those who in any way help forward our thought about ethics are working for the coming of peace and prosperity in the world. They are engaged in the higher politics, and the higher national economics." His ethical philosophy is based on reverence for life and the will-to-live which affirm both life and the world, and through activity then produce values. The thinking person feels the need to "give to every will-to-live the same reverence for life that he gives to his own. He experiences that other life in his own. He accepts as being good: to preserve life, to promote life, to raise to its highest value life which is capable of development; and as being evil: to destroy life, to injure life, to repress life which is capable of development." This universal ethic widens to include all that lives, and it seeks to relieve all suffering. One joins in the mysterious infinite will of all Being which acts for life through the person, giving meaning to existence from within outwards. To attain peace the ethic of reverence for life must be applied to the state so that collective interests will not overshadow the human feelings of empathy and cause interpersonal conflicts. The illusions of national interests must be criticized and replaced by moral and spiritual values, by concern for humanity as a whole.

In a world of violence Schweitzer still believed that truth, love, peacefulness, meekness, and kindness can overcome all violence. When a sufficient number with purity of heart, strength and perseverance think and live out the thoughts of love, truth, and peace, then the world will be theirs. Violence produces its own limitations, but kindness works simply and effectively without straining relations. A question Schweitzer posed was whether the spiritual will be strong and create world history or be weak and suffer world history. He believed that we will either realize the

Kingdom of God or perish, and the Kingdom of God begins in our hearts.

Schweitzer returned to Africa in 1924 and spent most of the next four decades working there. Occasionally he visited Europe, and in 1934 he vowed never to enter Nazi Germany. He was in Lambaréné throughout World War II. Hearing of V-E Day he quoted Lao Tzu's teaching that the victors ought not to rejoice in the murder of war but rather mourn as at a funeral. Following the war Schweitzer expressed concerns about the danger of nuclear war. He said that Africans could solve their own problems if the "civilized" nations of Europe and America did not blow up themselves and Africa first. In 1953 he was given the Nobel Peace prize; he used the money for a building at the Leper Village he had established in Lambaréné.

In 1955 he corresponded with Albert Einstein concerning atomic weapons and the hazardous tests of atomic bombs. He also conferred with Bertrand Russell on the same problem. In April 1954 Schweitzer had suggested that the protest against the H-bomb should be initiated by scientists.

Hoping for a statement by the reknowned Schweitzer on the nuclear weapons issue, Norman Cousins traveled to Lambaréné to discuss the idea with the aging but vital doctor. Schweitzer said he was always reluctant to make public statements, preferring instead to make his life his argument. However, because of the overwhelming importance of the issue, Schweitzer agreed to consider it. The result was a series of three radio broadcasts from Oslo, Norway in 1958 and a letter to President Eisenhower.

In the first broadcast Schweitzer called for the renunciation of nuclear tests. He explained to the general public the harmful medical effects of radiation in the bones and blood and how this continues for generations causing birth defects. He referred to the declaration that was signed by 9,235 scientists throughout the world and given to the Secretary General of the United Nations by Linus Pauling in January 1958. This, he stated, refutes the propaganda that scientists do not agree on the dangers of radiation. He criticized the concept of "a permissable amount of radiation." Permitted by whom? he asked. He appealed especially to women to raise their voices against the nuclear tests that cause deformed babies. He asked why international law and the United Nations have not done anything about this. He cited the Soviet tests in Siberia and the American tests at Bikini Atoll that contaminated the Pacific Ocean and Japan. Mankind is imperiled by the tests. "Mankind insists that they stop, and has every right to do so."

The second talk discussed the danger of an atomic war. Schweitzer recounted the first decade of the nuclear arms race and concluded that as a result of the arms buildup neither side could be victorious in an atomic war. "Those who conduct an atomic war for freedom will die, or end their lives miserably. Instead of freedom they will find destruction." Missiles equipped with H-bombs have radically changed the situation. The United States and the Soviet Union threaten each other from a distance, and there is the danger of their war occurring on European soil. The United States is arming countries which may use the weapons for defense against the Soviet Union which in turn might defend itself. These countries include Turkey and key nations in the Middle East where both the U.S. and U.S.S.R. seek alliances by giving financial and military aid. Conflicts between these smaller countries could endanger the peace of the world. The technology required and the short time intervals involved mean that war could originate from a mere incident or even an error. He pointed out that these quick decisions are being "entrusted to an electronic brain" which may become faulty. He criticized America for terrifying her opponent "to maintain peace" and for attempting to pressure NATO countries into acquiring weapons in spite of adverse public opinion. "The theory of peace through terrifying an opponent by a greater armament can now only heighten the danger of war." He supported the recent proposal to establish an atom-free zone in Europe and re-affirmed the public opinion in Europe "that under no circumstances is Europe to become a battlefield for an atomic war between the Soviet Union and the United States."

In the third broadcast Schweitzer proposed negotiations at the highest level for complete nuclear disarmament with international verification. There is no justification for nuclear weapons or tests, because they threaten the health and very existence of mankind. He suggested that America withdraw its forces from Europe, for the Europeans, East and West, must learn to get along with each other. The Soviet Union should also agree to reduce her army and agree not to attack Germany. We must rid ourselves of the paralyzing mistrust of our adversaries and approach each other "in the spirit that we are human beings, all of us." He sees two choices: one is a mad atomic-arms race with the danger of an unavoidable atomic war; the other is a mutual renunciation of nuclear weapons in the hope that we can manage to live in peace. Because the first is hopeless, we must risk the second.

Albert Schweitzer continued his medical work until he died at the age of ninety. Even in 1965, his last year, he was deeply upset about the Vietnam War, the tensions in the Middle East, and relations between the United States, Russia, and China. He died in Africa among the people he had served.

18

The Pacifism of Bertrand Russell and A. J. Muste

"Life and hope for the world
are to be found only in the deeds of love."

Bertrand Russell

"Either man will abolish war, or war will abolish man."

Bertrand Russell

"War can only be abolished
by the establishment of a world government."

Bertrand Russell

"The time has come, or is about to come,
when only large-scale civil disobedience,
which should be nonviolent,
can save the populations from the universal death
which their governments are preparing for them."

Bertrand Russell

"For love of domination we must substitute equality;
for love of victory we must substitute justice;
for brutality we must substitute intelligence;
for competition we must substitute cooperation.
We must learn to think of the human race as one family."

Bertrand Russell

"The survival of democracy
depends on the renunciation of violence
and the development of nonviolent means
to combat evil and advance the good."

A. J. Muste

"Only the nonviolent can apply therapy to the violent."

A. J. Muste

"There is no way to peace; peace is the way."

A. J. Muste

One of the greatest philosophers of the twentieth century, Bertrand Russell, was an active pacifist who spent considerable energy working for world peace, especially in his eighties and nineties. Bertrand Russell was born in England on May 18, 1872, and he died on February 2, 1970. Both of his parents died while he was a small child, and he was raised by his grandmother Russell. Bertrand was well educated; he was an outstanding student at Trinity College, Cambridge. In addition to his expertise in mathematics and philosophy he studied and lectured on economics and political science. Although he believed that the intellect maintained his sanity, he considered the emotions and passions fundamental in human life. He married four times. His skeptical attitudes and questioning of authority and popular tradition made him seem scandalous to many people.

Russell earned his reputation as a distinguished thinker by his work in mathematics and logic. In 1903 he published *The Principles of Mathematics* and by 1913 he and Alfred North Whitehead had published the three volumes of *Principia Mathematica*. Although Russell was an analytic rationalist all of his life, he did have a highly significant mystical experience in 1901 which influenced his values for the rest of his life. In his *Autobiography* he described what happened.

> Suddenly the ground seemed to give way beneath me, and I found myself in quite another region. Within five minutes I went through some such reflections as the following: the loneliness of the human soul is unendurable; nothing can penetrate it except the highest intensity of the sort of love that religious teachers have preached; whatever does not spring from this motive is harmful, or at best useless; it follows that war is wrong, that a public school education is abominable, that the use of force is to be deprecated, and that in human relations one should penetrate to the core of loneliness in each person and speak to that.

The usually skeptical Russell called it a "mystical illumination;" for a while he felt he could sense people's inmost thoughts; he became closer to his friends; he changed from an imperialist to a pacifist and sided with the Boers against Britain; for a time his analytic mind was swept away by ecstatic feelings about beauty, an intense interest in children, and the desire to found a philosophy, as the Buddha had done, to make human life more endurable.

During the first world war Russell's pacifism challenged British society. In July 1914 he collected signatures from fellow professors for a statement urging England to remain neutral in the imminent war. When the British were swept into the war and 90% of the population favored the fighting and killing, Russell was horrified and reassessed his views of human nature. In a letter to the London *Nation* for August 15 he criticized the pride of patriotism which promotes mass murder.

Bertrand Russell was not an absolute pacifist. He explained, "The use of force is justifiable when it is ordered in accordance with law by a neutral authority, in the general interest and not primarily in the interest of one of the parties to the quarrel." One solution, then, was for an international organization backed up by force to keep the peace. Another solution he suggested was passive resistance. If this was intelligently adopted by the whole nation with as much courage and discipline as was being shown in the war, then the national life could be better protected with far less carnage and waste.

In 1916 Russell began to work for the No Conscription Fellowship, and he became its chairman when all of the original committee had gone to prison. He wrote a leaflet to defend the case of Ernest Everett who had refused military service. When six men were arrested for distributing the leaflet, Russell wrote to *The Times* declaring he was its author. Russell was accused of hampering recruiting, and as his own attorney he explained that the case of a conscientious objector could hardly influence someone who is considering volunteering. He cited the English tradition of liberty, but he was convicted nonetheless. When he refused to pay the fine, the authorities preferred confiscating some of his possessions to putting him in prison. This conviction, however, prevented him from getting a passport to visit America. Russell felt that the more policemen and officials they could occupy with the innocent work of monitoring their pacifist activities, the less men would be available for the "official business of killing each other."

After Wilson's re-election in 1916, Russell wrote an open letter to the President which Katherine Dudley smuggled across the Atlantic. He appealed to the United States Government to make peace between the European Governments. He wrote, "If the German Government, as now seems likely, would not only restore conquered territory, but also give its adherence to the League to Enforce Peace or some similar method of settling disputes without war, fear would be allayed, and it is almost certain that an offer of mediation from you would give rise to an irresistible movement in favour of negotiations."

Russell's speeches to munition workers in South Wales were inaccurately reported by detectives, and the War Office forbade Russell from entering prohibited areas. In January 1918 an article by Russell appeared in a little weekly newspaper called *The Tribunal* suggesting that American soldiers were likely to be used as strike-breakers in England, since they had been employed in that way in the United States. This statement was backed up by a Senate Report. For this, Russell was sentenced to prison for six months. He spent the uninterrupted time cheerfully writing.

During the war Russell published several books on politics, war, and peace. *Principles of Social Reconstruction* was released in America as *Why Men Fight*. In this work Russell begins with the idea that the passions of war must be controlled, not by thought alone, but by the passion and desire to think clearly. Reason by itself is too lifeless. Wars can be prevented by a positive life of passion. Impulse must not be weakened but directed "towards life and growth rather than towards death and decay." Russell suggests that the excessive discipline of impulse not only exhausts vitality but often results in impulses of cruelty and destruction; this is why militarism is bad for national character. He recommends therefore active pacifism with the impulse and passion to overcome the impulses of war. Great courage and passion are necessary to face the onslaught of the hostile public opinion of a nation. Three forces for life are love, constructiveness, and joy. There must be strong action to assure international justice by a "Parliament of the nations." War can be prevented if the great powers firmly determine that peace shall be preserved. They could establish diplomatic methods to settle disputes and educational systems to teach the horrors of killing rather than admiration for war. Peace can only be permanently maintained by a world federation with the civil functions of a state — legislative, administrative, and judicial — and an international military force. This authority would legislate, adjudicate, and enforce international laws, but would not interfere with the internal affairs of nations. Pragmatically he suggests that at any given time we ought to support the best direction of movement available in the situation. This direction can be determined by applying the two principles of liberty and reverence. In other words, the freedom of individuals and communities ought to be encouraged, but not at the expense of others.

Russell replied to the War Office's restriction of his movement in the book *Justice in War Time*. He refused to surrender his spiritual liberty and declared that they could not prevent him from discussing political subjects, although they could imprison him under the Defense of the Realm Act. In the book he delineates the evils of war: the young men killed and maimed, the atrocities to non-combatants, the poverty of economic and social conditions, and the spiritual evils of hatred, injustice, falsehood, and conflict. He traces the theory of non-resistance held by Quakers and Tolstoy, and he imagines what might happen if England would be giving up its Empire and therefore could not be resistance and non-cooperation with the invaders as a means of defense. First there would be no justification at all for aggression. Englad would be giving up its Empire and therefore could not be accused of oppressing anyone. Even if Germans did invade, what could they do if all the officials refused to cooperate? Would they really shoot or imprison them all? If the population refused to obey any German orders, they would not learn German nor serve in the army nor even work to pay taxes or supply products. Russell notes that this would require courage and discipline. The most the Germans could do would be to take away the Empire and withhold food while demanding tribute. For Russell, the Empire is not a source of pride, and its self-governing parts could do the same thing. Demanding tribute is like the highwayman who says, "Your money or your life." Just as a reasonable man would hand over his money rather than be shot, a reasonable nation ought to give tribute rather than resist by force of arms. Primarily the rich would lose by this, because the poor would have to retain enough to be able to work and supply the means of tribute. It is unlikely that this tribute would be more than the cost of fighting the war. Many deaths and the moral degradation of war would be avoided. Russell suggests that it takes more courage and discipline to practice non-resistance than it does to kill out of fear. Thus militarism is due to "cowardice, love of dominion, and lust for blood." Even though non-resistance is a better defense than fighting, the more likely solution to the threat of war is the establishment of world government.

In *Political Ideals* Russell discusses the need for an international government to secure peace in the world by means of effective international law. Just as police are needed to protect private citizens from the use of force, so an international police can prevent the lawless use of force by states. The benefit of having law rather than international anarchy will give the international government a respected authority so that states will no longer feel free to use aggression. Then a large international force will become unnecessary.

Roads to Freedom includes a section where Russell points out the capitalistic factors which promote war. First is the desire of finance to exploit the resources of undeveloped countries. Second, large newspapers require capital and promote capitalistic interests. Third, capitalists like power and expect to command others. Nevertheless Russell does not recommend abolishing capitalism as a means to peace. However, he does recommend abolishing the private ownership of land and capital as one necessary step toward peace. Writing in 1918 he supports the idea of the League of Nations and international cooperation. He asserts, "No idea is so practical as the idea of the brotherhood of man." Again he emphasizes the need for a world government and national disarmament. In 1923 he wrote, "Without a world-government it will be impossible to preserve civilization for another hundred years." He declared the fundamental principle that the rights of a nation against humanity are no more absolute than the rights of an individual against the community.

While visiting China in 1920 Russell fell ill and was treated by John Dewey. Dewey was moved by a statement Russell made while he was delirious — "We must make a plan for peace." In

1922 Russell was intending to go to a Congress in Italy, but Mussolini informed the organizers of the Congress that, while no harm was to be done to Russell, any Italian who spoke to him was to be assassinated. Naturally Russell decided to avoid the country he felt Mussolini was defiling. In 1931 Russell applauded Einstein's statement recommending that pacifists refuse military service. Like Einstein, Russell decided not to adhere to absolute pacifism in the face of the Nazi threat.

Russell published *Which Way to Peace?* in 1936. He criticized isolationism and encouraged international law and government with an international armed force to prevent war. He could not imagine Hitler, Mussolini, or Stalin voluntarily renouncing national power. He also felt that England would not consent until after the disaster of war and that the United States would be reluctant unless Washington was in control. He cites Denmark as a successful example of national pacifism. Russell indicates that the three obstacles to disarmament are fear, pride, and greed.

The development of nuclear weapons caused Bertrand Russell deep concern. In November 1945 he gave a speech in the House of Lords warning that atomic weapons were going to be made more destructive and cheaper. Understanding nuclear physics he explained how a hydrogen bomb with much more explosive force could work. He predicted that soon the Russians would have bombs as destructive as those of the United States. He recommended that nuclear weapons be under international control, and he supported the Baruch Plan for an International Atomic Development Authority. Such great danger did he see if Russia and other nations developed atomic weapons that during this period when the United States was the only nuclear power he advocated that the U.S. ought to force the Russians to accept a world government under American leadership, even by going to war against Russia if necessary. He believed that the only cause worth fighting for was world government. He compared this policy to the alternative of waiting until the Russians had atomic bombs and choosing between a nuclear war and submission. Russell never liked Communism, but his anti-Communism was moderated with the death of Stalin. McCarthyism's restriction of civil liberties and the Bikini test in 1954 gradually led Russell to consider the United States a greater threat to unleash nuclear war than the Russians.

In 1950 Bertrand Russell was given the Nobel Prize for Literature. The last twenty years of his life were primarily devoted to warnings about the nuclear danger, advocacy of world government, and the active work of peacemaking and protesting about policies of war. He believed that world government was the only alternative to the disaster of nuclear war. People and nations must become willing to submit to international law. *New Hopes for a Changing World* is an optimistic view of how to solve world problems. He suggests that happiness depends on harmony with other people. The problem in forming a world government is that the nations are not yet willing to give it enough power to be effective. Yet war is inevitable as long as different sovereign states try to settle their disagreements by the use of armed force. Russell expressed the hope that if the West with its superior strength does not go to war, after a while the Russians may become less suspicious and begin to have friendly relations, which eventually could open the way to world government. Then both countries could be spared the expense of armaments, could benefit from reciprocal trade, and could escape the threat of nuclear destruction.

On March 1, 1954 the Bikini test of the H-bomb made it clear that this weapon is about one thousand times more powerful than the A-bomb. The radioactive fallout also proved to be deadly. Russell suggested that all fissionable raw material be owned by an international authority. International inspectors ought to make sure that no nation or individual has access to fissionable raw material. On December 23, 1954 Russell made a broadcast over the B.B.C. on "Man's Peril." He spoke not as a Briton or European but as a human being. He recommended that some neutral countries form a commission of experts to report on the destructive effects of a war using hydrogen bombs and that they submit this report to the Governments of the Great Powers so that they could agree that a world war could not serve the purpose of any of them. Russell asked everyone to remember their humanity and forget the rest so that a new Paradise would open instead of the way to universal death. Russell followed this address by drafting a statement for scientists to sign. He sent it to Einstein and was disappointed when he heard the news of Einstein's death. However, as one of his last acts, the great scientist had sent Russell a letter agreeing to sign. This Russell-Einstein Manifesto was also signed by a Communist scientist and several Nobel Prize-winners.

The Parliamentary Association for World Government in August 1955, invited representatives from every country, including four from the USSR. Russell moved a resolution urging "the governmnts of the world to realize and to acknowledge publicly that their purposes cannot be furthered by world war." Russell addressed an open letter to Eisenhower and Khrushchev in November 1957, asking that they make an agreement with each other on some points in which the interests of Russia and America are the same. Russell proposed the following: first, since the continued existence of the human race is paramount, neither side should incite war by trying for world dominion; second, the diffusion of nuclear weapons to other countries must be stopped; third, lessening hostility could lead to immense savings on armament expenditures; and fourth, by respecting each other's rights and using argument instead of force, fears of collective death could be diminished.

Bertrand Russell was one of the main organizers of the Pugwash Conferences of Scientists. At the first meeting in 1957 three committees were formed — one on the hazards of atomic energy, one on the control of nuclear weapons, and one on the social responsibilities of scientists. One of the achievements of the Pugwash movement was the eventual agreement on at least a partial Test-ban Treaty. Russell considered this only a slight mitigation of the dangers. Russell was also the President of the Campaign for Nuclear Disarmament (CND) which worked for the unilateral disarmament of Britain and the expulsion of U.S. bases from her soil.

Russell was also expressing his views on television in 1959 and in the books *Common Sense and Nuclear Warfare* and *Has Man a Future?* Nuclear warfare imperils mankind as a whole and therefore is to be treated like an epidemic and not be entangled in the conflicts of power politics. As a mathematician Russell knew that as long as nuclear war is a possibility its probability over time is increased. He quotes Linus Pauling's estimates of the hundreds of thousands of birth defects and embryonic and neo-natal deaths likely if tests are continued. The steps toward peace include the abolition of nuclear tests, the solving of differences without the threat of war, complete disarmament of nuclear weapons and a reduction of conventional forces, appointment of a Conciliation Committee with representatives from the powers and neutrals, the prohibition of foreign troops on any territory, and the establishment of a Federal International Authority with armed force to prevent war. Russell cautions that the armed force should be in units of mixed nationalities and under the command of officers from neutral countries. A federal constitution would leave the nations autonomous in regard to their own internal affairs. The international court must have the same authority as national courts. To those who fear the tyranny of a world government Russell responds that there would be more real freedom in the world under effective law and that in large modern governments it is fairly easy to maintain civilian control over the military. Technical advances have not only made international anarchy infinitely more dangerous, but also the facility of world cooperation is now more available. Eventually, for the sake of a stable world, greater economic equality and opportunity must be granted to the poorer peoples of the world. Education ought to be global in scope and perspective. Also the increase of population must be brought under control. Peace movements in every country ought to work together in spite of minor differences.

At the age of 88 Russell came to believe that a more radical strategy was needed, and he resigned from the CND to begin to plan actions of civil disobedience through the Committee of 100. A sit-down demonstration took place at a U.S. Polaris Base in which 20,000 people attended a rally and 5,000 sat down and risked arrest. On August 6, 1961 ("Hiroshima Day") they met at Hyde Park, and Russell illegally used a microphone. He was arrested and convicted of inciting the public to civil disobedience;

his sentence was commuted to one week. Russell wrote eloquent leaflets and gave speeches for these and other demonstrations urging that the seriousness of nuclear peril justified non-violent civil disobedience against the offending governments which are "organizing the massacre of the whole of mankind."

In October and November of 1962 Bertrand Russell acted as a peacemaker in two very serious international crises, even though he was only a private citizen. When President Kennedy ordered the naval blockade of Cuba to stop any Russian ship from carrying missiles to the island, Russell issued a press statement, which began, "It seems likely that within a week you will all be dead to please American madmen." Russell hoped there would be large demonstrations of protest, and noted that the most impressive was in New York where Michael Scott and A.J. Muste spoke to ten thousand. On October 23 Russell sent a telegram to Kennedy, calling his action "desperate" and a "threat to human survival" without justification and pleading that he end the madness. To Khrushchev he telegraphed an appeal that he not be provoked but seek condemnation of U.S. action through the United Nations. On the next day Premier Khrushchev publicized a long letter in reply to Mr. Russell assuring him that the Soviet government would not be reckless as the Americans had been in their pre-election excitement. Russell then telegraphed Khrushchev thanking him for his "courageous stand for sanity" and asking him to hold back the ships so that the Americans could come to an agreement. He also telegraphed Kennedy to urge him to negotiate. Khrushchev ordered some ships to turn away and allowed others to be inspected; Russell praised the Soviet Premier for this magnanimous, unilateral act. In another press statement Russell argued that the U.S. blockade was illegal and immoral even though he believed nuclear bases to be intolerable in Cuba or *anywhere*. How would America respond if the Russians or Chinese blockaded Formosa?

Khrushchev offered to dismantle the nuclear bases in Cuba if the United States would guarantee that it would not invade Cuba. This Cuban fear was obviously valid, since the U.S. had already tried to invade once at the Bay of Pigs. When Kennedy cabled Russell about the "secret Soviet missiles" and the Russian "burglars," he pointed out that they had not been secret, that even if they had been long-range, which they were not, the U.S. and U.S.S.R. already had enough long-range missiles and submarines to destroy each other, and that the Russians were not burglars any more than Americans in Britain and Western Europe; actually the Americans were contemplating "burglary." Russell wired Kennedy, asking him to "accept United Nations inspection of bases and to offer bases in Turkey in exchange." This would show America's stand for peace. He cabled Dr. Castro, requesting that he accept the dismantling and U.N. inspection in exchange for the pledge not to be invaded. Russell sent a long letter to Khrushchev, suggesting further steps toward peace, such as the abandonment of the Warsaw Pact. He telegraphed U.N. Secretary General U Thant, asking him if he would arbitrate and inspect bases. Castro wanted U Thant to mediate in Cuba, but the U.S. refused to discuss the Guantanamo base or accept U.N. inspectors of Florida camps. In the face of U.S. intransigence to trading bases in Turkey, Russell telegraphed Castro and Khruschchev, urging them to dismantle the bases, since even the insane American blackmail is preferrable to catastrophe. Although he was no lover of Communism, in this instance Russell commended Khrushchev for his wisdom and courage and criticized Kennedy for violating the U.N. Charter and perverting the Monroe Doctrine into the idea that if the U.S. does not like the form of government of a Western Hemisphere state and is threatening to attack it, then no outside power ought to try to help it.

In November 1962 Russell was similarly involved in mediating the border dispute between China and India. In numerous telegrams to Nehru and Chou En-lai, Russell urged a cease-fire and withdrawal so that negotiation and arbitration could settle the conflict. He also urged President Sukarno of Indonesia and U Thant to help mediate. In this situation India, which as a neutral nation had so often pleaded for peaceful relations, seemed to be overcome by war hysteria, and thus Russell found that the nation for which he had the most sympathy again was being the most unreasonable. This time Chou En-lai exercised wisdom and thanked Russell for his peacemaking efforts.

Reflecting on these two crises, Russell reiterated the danger of brinksmanship and the need for nuclear disarmament, since nuclear weapons only offer the options of complete submission or annihilation. The value of an unarmed and reasonable mediator made it easier for Khrushchev and others to make concessions without damaging their pride as much. Russell hoped that these crises might help discredit the Western belief that all Communists are wicked and all anti-Communists are virtuous. These situations and many others indicate the need for world government and strong international law so that disputes can be peacefully decided in courts.

The Bertrand Russell Peace Foundation was formed in 1963. He worked to free political prisoners in over forty countries. Russell began publishing articles criticizing the unofficial war in Vietnam. He explained how the French, Japanese, British, and Americans had prevented the Vietnamese people from obtaining their independence for the sake of imperialism and capitalistic exploitation. He described the atrocities that had been perpetrated by puppet governments of the West and American "advisors." By mid-1963 there were "160,000 dead; 700,000 tortured and maimed; 400,000 imprisoned; 31,000 raped; 3,000 disembowelled with livers cut out while alive; 4,000 burned alive; 1,000 temples destroyed; 46 villages attacked with poisonous chemicals;" and eight million villagers in 6,000 concentration camps. He felt the time for protest was overdue. By 1965 the numbers had increased and in a speech criticizing the British Labour Party's foreign policy Russell tore up his Labour Party membership card. He complained that visas the Peace Foundation had requested for three members of the National Liberation Front (NLF) had been refused. Russell backed up his vituperative criticism of U.S. policies with numerous facts and figures. He appealed to Americans to understand and overcome the cruel rulers who had taken control of the U.S. government. In 1966 he gave four reasons why the United States must be compelled to withdraw from Vietnam. First, the U.S. war crimes in Vietnam had been amply documented. Second, the U.S. had no right to be there; only a puppet ruler and a few ambitious Vietnamese generals wanted them there. Third, U.S. claims of "halting aggression" were absurd since the Geneva agreements had arranged for unification of Vietnam through election, which the U.S. had blocked. Fourth, the U.S. must not be encouraged to think that aggression pays. On May 24, 1966 Bertrand Russell spoke over NLF radio to American soldiers to explain to them the injustice of their involvement. Since the U.S. was continuing to drop three million pounds of bombs daily on North Vietnam, Russell called for an international War Crimes Tribunal in keeping with the principles of the Nuremburg trials. The Tribunal convened in November 1966 to announce that it would prepare evidence in the following five areas: "1. the crime of aggression, involving violation of international treaties; 2. the use of experimental weapons, such as gas and chemicals; 3. the bombing of hospitals, sanatoria, schools, dykes and other civilian areas; 4. the torture and mutilation of prisoners; 5. the pursuit of genocidal policies, such as forced labour camps, mass burials and other techniques of extermination in the South." Distinguished individuals from various countries agreed to join the Tribunal. The War Crimes Tribunal met in Sweden and Denmark and became independent of the Bertrand Russell Peace Foundation. Russell was now 95. He continued to work for peace to the end, and his last political statement was a condemnation of Israel's aggression sent to the International Conference of Parliamentarians in Cairo in February 1970.

Abraham Johannes Muste was born in Zeeland of the Netherlands on January 8, 1885; his family brought him to the United States at the age of six and raised him in Michigan as a Calvinist. He graduated from Union Theological Seminary in New York in 1909, and married that year. He was ordained a minister, but during World War I his pacifist convictions and ideas led to his resignation.

Moving to Boston in 1918 Muste formed a Comradeship of pacifists and began to observe the labor situation at the Lawrence textile mills. He felt that during the war the pacifists had not risked their lives, but the strike was an opportunity to see if nonviolence really works. Muste raised money for the strikers and was soon made the executive secretary of the strike committee for 30,000 strikers. A.J. placed himself at the head of the picket line and was beat to exhaustion by the police and arrested. Several weeks into the strike the police tried to provoke violence by lining up machine guns and having a labor spy urge the strikers to overcome them. Muste suggested that the strikers take the following courageous action:

> I told them, in line with the strike committee's decision, that to permit ourselves to be provoked into violence would mean defeating ourselves; that our real power was in our solidarity and our capacity to endure suffering rather than to give up the right to organize; that no one could "weave wool with machine guns;" that cheerfulness was better for morale than bitterness and that therefore we would smile as we passed the machine guns and the police on the way from the hall to the picket lines around the mill. I told the spies, who were sure to be in the audience, to go and tell the police and the mill managements that this was our policy.

This speech was greeted by cheers, and they went out, laughing and singing. Later Muste's room was broken into by a strong-arm squad, but he was not there. A colleague of his was taken out into the country, beat terribly, and left senseless in a ditch. After fifteen weeks the workers were weakening. Muste and the leaders successfully urged them to stay out for a week longer, but decided they would not pressure them after that. Muste was leaving town to report their failure to the union headquarters when he was contacted by management to arrange a settlement granting the strikers' demands.

Muste served as general secretary of the Amalgamated Textile Workers for over two years. Strikes occurred somewhere almost every week. From 1921 to 1933 he was the educational director of Brookwood Labor College. During the Depression he worked with the labor movement, the Unemployed Leagues, the Workers Party, the sit-down strikes, and the forming of the C.I.O. Muste helped start the Conference for Progressive Labor Action (CPLA) which offered a radical alternative to the Communist Party. In 1936 he helped organize a strike of the Goodyear Tire workers in Akron, Ohio, which was the first time the sit-in tactic was used in the American labor movement. Also in 1936 A.J. gave up his Trotskyism and returned to Christian pacifism for the rest of his life, saying that God is love and that "love is the central thing in the universe." Love, he felt, must be carried into every aspect of family life, race relations, labor movement, political activity, and international relations.

In 1940 A.J. Muste published *Non-violence in an Aggressive World* outlining a Christian pacifist approach to revolution in a war-torn world. He describes the interrelationships of the three revolutionary reform movements to which he was committed in the fields of religion, economics, and politics — namely Christianity, socialism, and democracy. He urges a pacifist revolution which will enlighten minds and redirect wills. With unity and solidarity among the workers and using nonviolent methods, Muste predicts there will be less economic and social dislocation than in most revolutions. He criticizes the totalitarian repression, terrorism, and conformity of some post-revolutionary regimes, and he calls instead for democratic and brotherly life. Although he considers struggling against injustice by any means to be nobler than cowardice, Muste's experience in the labor movement led him to believe that violence was always self-defeating. "The oppressed will make surer and faster progress if they eschew violence and depend, as they do mainly depend in their organizing and strike activities, on their solidarity, courage, capacity for suffering and sacrifice, and on non-cooperation where injustice becomes extreme." Instead of using national armies, Muste saw the need for an international police force. A political federation built on fair economic arrangements will be held together by mutual benefits, making armies unnecessary. He points out that there is a necessary connection between democracy and nonviolence; when external force is used, freedom is lost. Racism and nationalism which promote war are destructive to democracy, corrupting the external and internal relations of a country. Imperialism in foreign policy likewise causes injustice and oppression at home as well as abroad through the "crushing burden of militarism and totalitarian war." Muste advocates unilateral disarmament, pointing out how reluctant people are to fight and kill in a war. How could they be led to slaughter a helpless population? "With much less effort than is required to put a nation on a war-basis, it could be organized to meet, confuse, and rout an invader with nonviolent noncooperation." He concludes that pacifism is based on love and fellowship and treating one's neighbor as oneself; our resources for living this life of love have hardly been tapped at all so far.

In an essay on "The World Task of Pacifism" in 1941 Muste declared that as long as people believe that war is a solution to social problems, then human resources will be devoted to "forging diabolically effective instruments of slaughter and destruction." Once this delusion has been dispelled, then a new order will be built. In another essay that year he suggested the following:

> Christian realism would lead us to renounce war preparation and war as obviously suicidal; to offer to surrender our own special privileges; to participate in lowering tariff walls, in providing access to basic resources on equitable terms to all peoples; to spend the billions we shall otherwise squander on war preparations, and war, for the economic rehabilitation of Europe and Asia, for carrying a great "offensive" of food, medicine, and clothing to the stricken peoples of the world; and to take our full share of responsibility for building an effective federal world government.

In 1942 Muste suggested that the United States enter into negotiations with all the nations in the war with the following proposals: 1) the U.S. will help build a federal world government; 2) the U.S. will invest billions for the economic rehabilitation of Europe and Asia; 3) "no attempt shall be made to fasten *sole* war-guilt on any nation or group of nations;" 4) subject nations such as India, Philippines, Puerto Rico, Denmark, Norway, France, Belgium, and Holland must be granted full self-determination; 5) "all peoples should be assured of equitable access to markets and to essential raw materials;" 6) to further democracy the U.S.

should provide decent housing, adequate medical and hospital service, and equal educational facilities for all its people, "including Negroes and Orientals;" 7) the U.S. must repudiate racism and call on Germany and other countries to do the same; and 8) drastic reduction of armaments by all nations should move all rapidly to an economy of peace.

As early as 1943 Muste recommended the use of nonviolent methods to bring an end to Jim Crow practices of racial discrimination. He was Executive Secretary of the Fellowship of Reconciliation (FOR) from 1940 until 1953 where he influenced civil rights leaders such as James Farmer and Bayard Rustin who were FOR staff members. In 1942 they founded the Congress of Racial Equality (CORE). Martin Luther King, Jr. and others were also influenced by Muste's nonviolence philosophy and tactics. During the war he gave moral support to conscientious objectors, and in 1947 he sponsored a session of draft card burning. Muste refused to pay Federal income tax from 1948 on. After the war he completely rejected Communism, but during the McCarthy period Muste spoke out for the civil rights of Communists. He called for the cessation of hostilities in Korea, urged the United Nations to stop acting as a war agency, advocated that U.S. abandon war and adopt nonviolence, and promoted the spirit of pacifism.

Muste helped organize and participated in many direct action campaigns. In 1955 he joined Dorothy Day and others in refusing to take cover in a New York civil defense drill. On August 7, 1957 he participated in a vigil protesting nuclear weapons tests near Las Vegas, Nevada. The following year he was an advisor in the project of sailing the *Golden Rule* into a bomb-test area. He chaired the "Walk for Peace Committee" which included the American Friends Service Committee, *The Catholic Worker,* the Fellowship of Reconciliation, Peacemakers, the War Resisters League, and the Women's International League for Peace and Freedom. For the Committee for Nonviolent Action (CNVA) Muste coordinated the Omaha Action project and was arrested as one of the trespassers at the Mead Missile Base. He considered nuclear war politically irrational, morally indefensible, and a hideous atrocity. Even preparation for such a war is a

194

degradation of mankind. Neither the aims of Communism nor those of Christian democracy can be advanced or even salvaged after a nuclear war. To threaten the obliteration of an enemy people he referred to as an extreme mental sickness. The real enemy is war.

In December 1959 Muste traveled to Africa to help coordinate a protest against French nuclear bomb-tests in the Sahara. Meanwhile the Peace Walk had gone from San Francisco to Moscow. About 80,000 leaflets were distributed in the Soviet Union; the demonstrators spoke to meetings of several hundred people every night. Muste felt national barriers had been transcended in favor of a common humanity. In 1961 an experimental World Peace Brigade was formed at a conference in Beirut, Lebanon, under the direction of Muste, Michael Scott, and Jayaprakash Narayan. A training center for nonviolent action was established in Dar es Salaam, Tanzania. Muste hoped this was a beginning toward realizing Gandhi's concept of a world peace army *(Shanti sena)*. In the summer of 1962 the World Peace Brigade and others, such as the CNVA, CND, and the Committee of 100, sponsored the voyage of *Everyman III* to Leningrad to protest Soviet nuclear testing.

In the early Vietnam War era Muste was able to help bring together a broad-based coalition of groups to protest. He helped to establish the policy of refusing to accept the co-sponsorship of organizations that support war, military build-up, or violence, although any individual accepting nonviolent discipline could participate. In 1965 over 50,000 people paraded down Fifth Avenue in New York. Again in this war he suggested that the United States withdraw its forces and disarm. To young men facing conscription he always recommended "holy disobedience." In 1966 Muste met with anti-war Buddhist and Catholic leaders in Saigon. In January 1967 he met with Ho Chi Minh in Hanoi to try to find ways to end the war. Muste died seventeen days later. He was honored in New York at the Spring Mobilization to End the War in Vietnam march.

19

Martin Luther King and the Civil Rights Movement

"True peace is not merely the absence of tension;
it is the presence of justice."

Martin Luther King, Jr.

"With nonviolent resistance,
no individual or group need submit to any wrong,
nor need anyone resort to violence in order to right a wrong."

Martin Luther King, Jr.

"Unearned suffering is redemptive.
Suffering, the nonviolent resister realizes,
has tremendous educational and transforming possibilities."

Martin Luther King, Jr.

"The aftermath of nonviolence is reconciliation
and the creation of the beloved community."

Martin Luther King, Jr.

From 1956 until his tragic death in 1968 Martin Luther King, Jr. was the foremost leader in black Americans' nonviolent quest for civil rights and a better life. He was born on January 15, 1929 in Atlanta, Georgia and was named after his father who was a successful Baptist preacher. His father taught him self-respect in the face of racial discrimination. Martin started at Morehouse College in Atlanta when he was only 15, and he graduated four years later. Choosing the ministry over medicine and law he attended Crozer Theological Seminary in Pennsylvania for three years. While there he heard A.J. Muste lecture, and after hearing Mordecai Johnson lecture on Gandhi he went out and bought every book he could find on Gandhi and nonviolence. Martin had already read Thoreau's "Essay on Civil Disobedience" at Morehouse; he was so moved by the idea of refusing to cooperate with an evil system that he reread it several times. In his theological studies he leaned toward the social gospel of Walter Rauschenbusch. He read Marx and rejected his materialism and deprecation of individual freedom; however, he also questioned the materialism and injustices of capitalism.

In reading Gandhi, King realized that the love ethic of Jesus could go beyond individuals and be applied to the conflicts of racial groups and nations. He discovered the method for social reform in Gandhi's love force *(satyagraha)* and nonviolence. After being elected student body president and graduating first in his class at Crozer, King moved on to Boston University where he earned his Ph.D. in Theology. In 1953 he married Coretta Scott, a bright student of music, and they eventually had four children. Believing in the guidance of a personal God and equipped with the techniques of nonviolence, King accepted a pastorate in Montgomery, Alabama, hoping he could help his people achieve social justice.

King had only recently completed his doctoral dissertation and gotten settled in the Dexter Avenue Baptist Church when the issue of racial segregation on the public buses erupted in Montgomery. On May 17, 1954 the United States Supreme Court had declared, "Separate educational facilities are inherently unequal," and in 1955 the same Court ordered all public schools to be desegregated "with all deliberate speed." In Montgomery King had become active in the NAACP and in the integrated Alabama Council on Human Relations. In March 1955 a fifteen-year-old girl had been arrested for refusing to give up her seat to a white passenger on the bus. King was on the committee that protested this, but no action was taken. On December 1, 1955 Mrs. Rosa Parks felt her feet were too tired for her to stand up for a white man who had boarded after her. The bus driver ordered her to stand up and give her seat to the white man, but she refused. She was arrested and taken to the courthouse. From there she called E. D. Nixon who in turn made several calls. The Women's Political Council proposed a one-day boycott of the buses. The next morning, which was a Friday, Nixon called King, and he offered the Dexter Avenue Church as a meeting place for that night. Over forty black leaders showed up, and they agreed to boycott the buses on the following Monday and hold a mass meeting Monday night. Leaflets were mimeographed and distributed announcing these actions. Committees were organized, and alternative transportation was arranged. Recalling Thoreau's words about not cooperating with an evil system, King thought of the movement as massive non-cooperation.

The word spread, and on Monday morning the Montgomery buses were practically empty except for a few white passengers. Mrs. Parks was convicted that morning of disobeying the city's segregation ordinance and fined ten dollars and court costs. Her attorney appealed. That afternoon Dr. King was elected president of what became the Montgomery Improvement Association (MIA). The Holt Street Baptist Church had five thousand people standing outside listening to loudspeakers for the evening meeting. King spoke for the hearts of many when he declared that they were "tired of being segregated and humiliated." He affirmed that their only alternative was to protest for freedom and justice. Christian love and nonviolent principles provided the basis for his advice. He said, "No one must be intimidated to keep them from riding the buses. Our method must be persuasion, not coercion. We will only say to the people, 'Let your conscience be your guide.' " He concluded his speech, "If you will protest courageously, and yet with dignity and Christian love, future historians will say, 'There lived a great people — a black people — who injected new meaning and dignity into the veins of civilization.' This is our challenge and our overwhelming responsibility." Ralph Abernathy proposed three moderate demands which were unanimously approved at the mass meeting: 1) courteous treatment by bus operators; 2) passengers to be seated on a first-come, first-served basis with Negroes in the back and whites in the front; and 3) Negro bus drivers to be employed in predominantly Negro routes.

In his book *Stride Toward Freedom* King explains how Christian love and nonviolent methods guided the movement. In weekly meetings he would emphasize that the use of violence would be both impractical and immoral. "Hate begets hate; violence begets violence; toughness begets a greater toughness. We must meet the forces of hate with the power of love; we must meet physical force with soul force. Our aim must never be to defeat or humiliate the white man, but to win his friendship and understanding." Although to King nonviolence was a way of life, he was glad that the black people were willing to accept it as a method; he presented it simply as Christianity in action. In *Stride Toward Freedom* King elucidates six key points about the philosophy of nonviolence. First, it is not based on cowardice; although it may seem passive physically, it is spiritually active, requiring the courage to stand up against injustice. Second, nonviolence does not seek to defeat the opponent but rather to win his understanding to create "the beloved community." Third, the attack is directed at the evil not at the people who are doing the evil; for King the conflict was not between whites and blacks but between justice and injustice. Fourth, in nonviolence there is a willingness to accept suffering without retaliating. Fifth, not only is physical violence avoided but also spiritual violence; love replaces hatred. Sixth, nonviolence has faith that justice will prevail.

Meanwhile, to get people to work and back, black taxi companies had lowered their fares, car pools were arranged, and many people walked. However, the city prohibited the taxi companies from doing this business, threatened people with vagrancy and illegal-hitchhiking charges, and rumors spread that drivers might lose their licenses or insurance. King was arrested in January for driving 30 in a 25 mile-per-hour zone, even though he was driving very carefully since he was aware of being followed. The Kings' house was bombed; however, Coretta and a friend had escaped injury by moving quickly to the back of the house. Martin rushed home from his meeting, and a furious mob gathered outside. He calmed them down and advised them to put down their weapons and go home. He said, "We cannot solve this problem through retaliatory violence. We must meet violence with nonviolence . . . We must meet hate with love." When the mayor tried to speak, he was booed and threatened; but again King quieted the crowd. His presence and words had prevented a bloody riot. The Kings often received threatening phone calls, but even after the bomb blast, King would not allow a weapon in his house.

While King was away lecturing at Fisk University in Nashville, the Montgomery attorney began arresting MIA leaders for violating an old state law against boycotts. Against the advice of his father Martin returned to Montgomery to be placed under arrest. He was released on bail. On March 22 Judge Carter found eighty-nine defendants guilty. King was sentenced to pay a fine of $500 or serve 386 days hard labor. Appeals were filed. On June 4, 1956 a federal court held that bus segregation was unconstitutional. However, the city attorneys appealed to the Supreme Court. In November the city tried to ban the car pools. While they were in a Montgomery court on this charge, the Supreme Court affirmed the decision declaring Alabama's state and local laws requiring segregation on buses unconstitutional.

Meetings were held to prepare the people for integration of the buses. Training sessions in nonviolent techniques enabled "actors" to play out different roles before a critical audience which would discuss the results. Integrated bus suggestions were printed which recommended "complete nonviolence in word and action" and the admonition, "Be loving enough to absorb evil and understanding enough to turn an enemy into a friend." A few days before Christmas, after more than a year's boycott, the black ministers of Montgomery led the way in riding integrated buses. In January a few acts of terrorism occurred, but again King urged nonviolence and the way of the cross. After a few weeks the transportation systems had returned to normal with integrated buses.

The Montgomery success gave King national prominence. Along with Ralph Abernathy, Fred Shuttlesworth, and C.K. Steele, he formed the Southern Christian Leadership Conference (SCLC) with headquarters in Atlanta. He urged President Eisenhower to call for a White House Conference on Civil Rights. When the Eisenhower Administration failed to respond adequately, King organized a "Prayer Pilgrimage of Freedom" which drew thirty-seven thousand marchers to the Lincoln Memorial in Washington on May 17, 1957. King led the cry of blacks for the ballot so that they could participate more fully in the legislative process.

In 1958 *Stride Toward Freedom* came out calling for a militant and nonviolent mass movement. King suggests in this book that if they remain nonviolent, then public opinion will be magnetically attracted to them rather than to the instigators of violence. A nonviolent mass movement is power under discipline seeking justice. He summarizes his nonviolent intentions this way:

We will take direct action against injustice without waiting for other agencies to act. We will not obey unjust laws or submit to unjust practices. We will do this peacefully, openly, cheerfully because our aim is to persuade. We adopt the means of nonviolence because our end is a community at peace with itself. We will try to persuade with our words, but if our words fail, we will try to persuade with our acts. We will always be willing to talk and seek fair compromise, but we are ready to suffer, when necessary and even risk our lives to become witnesses to the truth as we see it.

He points out that nonviolence first affects the hearts of those committed to it, gives them greater self-respect and courage, and then it stirs the conscience of the opponents until reconciliation is achieved. In a world of ballistic missiles he declares, "Today the choice is no longer between violence and nonviolence. It is either nonviolence or nonexistence."

On Lincoln's birthday in 1958 twenty-one mass meetings were held simultaneously in key southern cities calling for "freedom now." In September King was arbitrarily arrested while in the Montgomery courthouse. He decided to refuse to pay bail or the fine. However, the officials preferred to pay his fine for him "to save the taxpayers the expense of feeding King for fourteen days."

While autographing copies of his book in New York, a psychotic woman stabbed King in the chest with a sharp letter-opener. He remained calm and waited for a surgeon to remove the knife-like weapon. Its point had been touching his aorta, and he was told that if he had merely sneezed he probably would have died.

In February 1959 Martin Luther King made a pilgrimage to India and returned even more confirmed in the principles of nonviolence. On the first of December King called for "a broad, bold advance of the southern campaign for equality." In 1960 student activists organized numerous sit-ins at lunch counters in order to end discrimination. King and James Lawson spoke on nonviolence at a meeting in Raleigh, North Carolina, and the Student Nonviolent Coordinating Committee (SNCC) was formed. King and thirty-six others were arrested for sitting at the lunch counter in Rich's Department Store in Atlanta. The judge sentenced King to six months hard labor. This was on October 25, and the election was only a few days away. President Eisenhower considered making a public statement, but he and Vice President Nixon decided not to comment. However, John Kennedy and his brother Robert made some phone calls urging King's release. Some say that this gesture helped Kennedy win the election over Nixon by a narrow margin.

King was elected chairman of the committee on the Freedom Rides in 1961. To protect the Freedom Riders from the onslaught of violence King requested Attorney General Robert Kennedy to send more federal marshalls. King explained, "The law may not be able to make a man love me, but it can keep him from lynching me." The Freedom Rides took the civil rights movement from the urban college campuses to the rural hamlets of the South.

King answered the call to help the movement in Albany, Georgia to desegregate public parks and other facilities. He and Ralph Abernathy were arrested in December 1961 for refusing to disperse. They were tried the following February and sentenced on July 10, 1962 to pay a fine or be imprisoned at hard labor for forty-five days. They chose prison. Again an anonymous person paid the fines. King then announced a civil disobedience campaign. However, when two thousand people threw rocks and bottles at the police, he called for a "Day of Penitence" and a week of prayer vigils. King, Abernathy, and Dr. Anderson were arrested at the first vigil. They spent two weeks in jail before the trial and then were given suspended sentences. A new demonstration was planned after their release, but this time the city obtained a federal injunction against the demonstration. Since the federal courts had always been their ally, King reluctantly cancelled the march. Many considered the Albany campaign a failure because it did not achieve desegregation, but King felt they learned tactical lessons and through increased voter registration began to affect elections more. Five percent of the black population had accepted nonviolence and had gone willingly to jail.

Fred Shuttlesworth of the Alabama Christian Movement for Human Rights had been working to desegregate Birmingham, but he was meeting much resistance. He requested the help of the SCLC, and in April 1963 after the elections involving Eugene "Bull" Connor they acted. Their organization had improved since Albany, and workshops on nonviolence and direct-action techniques were conducted. They began with sit-ins involving a few arrests each day. Mass meetings with talks on nonviolence were held each evening. Many volunteers came forward, and the movement grew into a nonviolent army. Each volunteer signed the following Commitment Card:

I hereby pledge myself — my person and body — to the nonviolent movement. Therefore I will keep the following ten commandments:

1. Meditate daily on the teachings and life of Jesus.
2. Remember always that the nonviolent movement in Birmingham seeks justice and reconciliation — not victory.
3. Walk and talk in the manner of love, for God is love.
4. Pray daily to be used by God in order that all men might be free.
5. Sacrifice personal wishes in order that all men might be free.
6. Observe with both friend and foe the ordinary rules of courtesy.
7. Seek to perform regular service for others and for the world.
8. Refrain from the violence of fist, tongue, or heart.
9. Strive to be in good spiritual and bodily health.
10. Follow the directions of the movement and of the captain on a demonstration.

King chose to postpone his own arrest so that he could speak to meetings in the black community; he appealed to ministers for help in the struggle to improve social conditions. On Saturday April 6, forty-two were arrested for "parading without a permit."

So far both sides were nonviolent, and they sang on their way to jail. The boycott of the downtown merchants was effective. There were kneel-ins at churches, sit-ins at the library, a march to the county building for voter registration, and the jails began to fill. They decided to disobey a state court injunction, because they felt Alabama was misusing the judicial process. Although most of the leaders wanted King to stay free in order to raise money, he asked Ralph Abernathy to go to jail with him. On Good Friday they were arrested, and King was put in solitary confinement. Coretta contacted President Kennedy to request help in improving King's jail conditions, and Harry Belafonte was able to raise fifty thousand dollars for bail bonds.

On scraps of paper Martin Luther King wrote his famous letter from Birmingham jail in which he responded to ministers' public charges that his actions were "unwise and untimely." He explains that he came to Birmingham because of the injustice there. They had gone through the four basic steps of a nonviolent campaign: collection of facts about injustice, negotiation, self-purification, and direct action. Just as Socrates had been an intellectual gadfly, he too must struggle against injustice. He states the hard truth, "We know through painful experience that freedom is never voluntarily given by the oppressor; it must be demanded by the oppressed." He quotes St. Augustine who said that "an unjust law is no law at all." Segregation is unjust because it damages the personality and creates false concepts of superiority and inferiority. To break an unjust law "openly, lovingly, and with a willingness to accept the penalty" is to express respect for real justice. He points out that what Hitler did in Germany was "legal," while aiding or comforting a Jew was "illegal." Their action does not create the tension; it merely brings to the surface the seething hidden tensions. Nonviolence offers a creative outlet for repressed emotions which might otherwise result in violence. If he is an extremist, then like Jesus he is an extremist for love.

After eight days King and Abernathy accepted bail. King then suggested that they enlist young people in the campaign. Andy Young sent some who were too young to the library to learn something. On May 2 over a thousand youths demonstrated and went to jail. King explains in his book *Why We Can't Wait* that all ages, sexes, races, and even the disabled can be accepted into a nonviolent army. When the jails were almost full, Bull Connor changed his tactics to violence, turning on the waterhoses, sending in police with their clubs, and releasing the police dogs. Moral indignation swept across the nation. On ·May 4 the Attorney General sent mediators to seek a truce. On May 10 an agreement was reached granting the major demands: desegregation of lunch counters, rest rooms, fitting rooms, and drinking fountains; upgrading and hiring of blacks on a nondiscriminatory basis; release of all jailed persons; and establishing communications between black and white leaders.

Segregationists reacted by bombing the house of Martin's brother A.D. King at midnight on Saturday in order to incite a riot. Followers of the movement sang "We Shall Overcome" to stop.the violence. The next day President Kennedy sent in three thousand federal troops. On May 20 the Supreme Court decided that demonstrations against segregated institutions are legal. Justice had triumphed.

King went on a speaking tour from Los Angeles to New York. In Detroit on June 23, 1963 he led 125,000 people on a Freedom Walk. To this crowd he spoke of nonviolence as a strong method of disarming the opponent. He declared, "If a man hasn't discovered something that he will die for, he isn't fit to live!"

At a conference with A. Philip Randolph and Roy Wilkins of the NAACP, John Lewis of SNCC, Dorothy Height of the National Council of Negro Women, James Farmer of CORE, and Whitney Young of the Urban League, they planned a march on Washington for "Jobs and Freedom" in order to put pressure on Congress to pass President Kennedy's Civil Rights Bill. Two hundred fifty thousand people, about a third of them white, congregated at the Lincoln Memorial on August 28, 1963. Randolph introduced King as the "moral leader of the nation." King began with his prepared speech about how America had given the Negro a bad check and they had come there to collect on the promises. The great crowd's response inspired him, and he put aside his text and began to speak of his dream of equality, brotherhood, and freedom — a dream where people are not judged by their skin color but by their character. He tolled the bell of freedom so that it would ring out all across the land.

When the assassination of President Kennedy was announced, King privately told Coretta that the same thing would happen to him because "this is a sick society." The following June King and Abernathy were arrested in St. Augustine, Florida. King explained how some people were trying to stop the movement by threatening them with physical death, but he responded, "If physical death is the price that I must pay to free my white brother and all my brothers and sisters from a permanent death of the spirit, then nothing can be more redemptive."

On July 2, 1964 King personally witnessed President Lyndon Johnson's signing of the Civil Rights law. King submitted an Economic Bill of Rights to the Democratic Party platform committee. He suggested that the disadvantaged who have been denied so long ought to receive something comparable to the GI Bill of Rights.

At age thirty-five Martin Luther King became the youngest person ever to receive a Nobel Prize. He accepted the prestigious award for peace on behalf of the Movement, saying it was "a profound recognition that nonviolence is the answer to the crucial political and racial questions of our time — the need for man to overcome oppression without resorting to violence."

In 1965 the push for voter registration was accelerated, and Selma, Alabama was selected as the most challenging target. Mass meetings were held there throughout January and February. On February first King and Abernathy led a march of 250 blacks and 15 whites to the courthouse where they all were arrested. On March 5 King spent two and a half hours with President Johnson urging him to expedite the Voting Rights Bill. On March 7 he announced a fifty-four mile march from Selma to Montgomery. Although Governor Wallace prohibited the march, King exhorted the people to stand up for what is right. SCLC strategy was for the leaders to avoid arrest in the early stages of a campaign. Thus King was not at the front of the march when they were met by Alabama troopers with gas masks, tear gas, clubs, horsemen with whips, and deputies with electric cattle prods. The brutal attack was cheered by whites on the sidelines.

King announced that he and Abernathy would lead another march. A federal injunction was issued against it, but King made a nationwide appeal for ministers and others to join them. This time they crossed the bridge before coming to the troopers. Fifteen hundred people prayed on the road, and then to avoid a violent confrontation King asked them to turn back. That night a white minister from Boston was murdered by four Klansmen in Selma. Demonstrations were held across the country, and four thousand religious leaders picketed the White House to push for the Voting Rights Bill. The evening of the funeral President Johnson gave his "We shall overcome" speech and made the Voting Rights Bill his top priority. The injunction against the march was lifted, and the President federalized the Alabama National Guard and sent troops to protect the marchers. On March 21 the march was successfully carried out, and when they got to Montgomery they were a crowd of fifty thousand. Again King's oratory lifted the people as he declared that they would not have to wait long for freedom because "no lie can live forever," because "you will reap what you sow," because "the arm of the moral universe is long but it bends toward justice," and because "mine eyes have seen the glory of the coming of the Lord." The Voting Rights Bill was signed on August 6, 1965.

Meanwhile problems were surfacing outside the South. In one night of rioting in the Watts section of Los Angeles more people were killed than in ten years of nonviolent demonstrations across the country. On June 6, 1966 James Meredith was shot while leading a march in Mississippi. King visited him in the hospital and took his place on the march. Stokely Carmichael and the Black Power advocates wanted to exclude whites, but King said he would withdraw. They agreed to keep the march interracial and nonviolent.

In January 1966 King had moved his family into a Chicago slum to begin a protest for better housing and economic conditions. Mayor Daly closed up City Hall, but like his namesake Martin Luther, King nailed his demands to the closed door. Finally, to avoid a violent confrontation Mayor Daly met with King, Archbishop Cody, Chicago Real Estate Board representatives, the Chicago Housing Authority, business and industrial leaders, and black leaders of Chicago and the SCLC. An open housing agreement was announced on August 26. An SCLC poverty and unemployment program called Operation Breadbasket was put under the leadership of Jesse Jackson.

King's conscience told him that he must speak out against the Vietnam War, even though the SCLC leaders asked him not to speak as SCLC President but as a private citizen. Many civil rights leaders considered his denunciation of Johnson's Vietnam policy a mistake. However, his wife Coretta, his former professor Harold de Wolf, A.J. Muste, and UN Ambassador Arthur Goldberg supported him for his courageous stand. In January 1967 in Los Angeles he declared, "The promises of the Great Society have been shot down on the battlefields of Vietnam . . . We must combine the fervor of the Civil Rights Movement with the peace movement." He spoke at the Spring Mobilization campaign organized by A.J. Muste. While in Geneva King called for an immediate negotiated settlement to the "immoral" war. At Riverside Church in New York he proposed a five-point peace program for Vietnam: an end to all bombing; a unilateral cease-fire to prepare for negotiation; curtailment of military build-ups throughout Southeast Asia; realistic acceptance of the National Liberation Front; and the withdrawal of all foreign troops from Vietnam in accordance with the 1954 Geneva agreement.

King believed that the root cause of both racial hatred and war was fear. He hoped that the greatest application of the nonviolent methods used in the civil rights movement would be for world peace. "Do we have the morality and courage required to live together as brothers and not be afraid?" he asked. War, he said, had become obsolete, but he knew the danger when he saw the leaders of nations preparing for war while talking peace. If we want mankind to survive, then we must find an alternative to war. Since modern weapons are calamitous, he suggested "that the philosophy and strategy of nonviolence become immediately a subject for study and for serious experimentation in every field of human conflict, by no means excluding the relations between nations." He had faith that we can end war and violence as long as we do not succumb to fear of the weapons we have created. He recommended that the United Nations consider using nonviolent direct action as an application of peaceable power. He prophesied that achieving disarmament and peace would depend on a spiritual re-evaluation. He warned that a nation which spends more money on military defense than on social programs is moving toward spiritual death. Ultimately there must be a world-wide fellowship based on unconditional love for all people.

In 1968 Martin Luther King was preparing a massive Poor People's Campaign for whites as well as blacks when he was called to Memphis to assist with a strike of the sanitation workers. Two thousand people at Clayborn Temple wanted to hear him speak. He declared his support for their cause, but then he began to reflect about the threats made against his life. He confessed that he would like a long life, but his main concern was to do God's will. He was glad that he had been to the mountaintop and seen the Promised Land. The next day, April 4, 1968, Martin Luther King, Jr. was shot and killed. He had already requested a simple eulogy two months before when he had said, "I'd like someone to mention that day that Martin Luther King, Jr., tried to give his life serving others. I'd like somebody to say that day that Martin Luther King, Jr., tried to love somebody. I want you to be able to say that day that I did try to feed the hungry. I want you to be able to say that day that I did try in my life to clothe the naked. I want you to say on that day that I did try in my life to visit those who were in prison. And I want you to say that I tried to love and serve humanity."

20
Lessons of Vietnam

"All the peoples on the earth are equal from birth;
all the peoples have a right to live, to be happy and free."

Declaration of Independence of the
Democratic Republic of Vietnam

"The United States must be compelled
to get out of Vietnam immediately and without conditions."

Bertrand Russell

"Let peace-minded persons and organizations
in every state of the United States
and in every country of the world
devise ways to call for an end to military intervention
in Vietnam as a first imperative step
to ending the threat of nuclear war
and bringing justice, freedom and peace to mankind."

A.J. Muste

"This war turns the clock of history back
and perpetuates white colonialism.
The greatest irony and tragedy of it all
is that our own nation which initiated so much
of the revolutionary spirit in this modern world
is now cast in the mold of being an arch anti-revolutionary."

Martin Luther King, Jr.

"I went to Vietnam, a hard charging Marine 2nd Lieutenant,
sure that I had answered the plea of a victimized people
in their struggle against communist aggression.
That belief lasted about two weeks.
Instead of fighting communist aggressors
I found that 90% of the time our military actions
were directed against the people of South Vietnam.
These people had little sympathy
or for that matter knowledge of the Saigon Government.
We are engaged in a war in South Vietnam
to pound a people into submission to a government
that has little or no popular support

among the real people of South Vietnam.
By real people I mean all those Vietnamese people
who aren't war profiteers or who have not sold out
to their government or the United States
because it was the easy and/or profitable thing to do."

letter to Senator Fulbright

"Obviously a major lesson of Vietnam
is that we must know ourselves better."

Daniel Ellsberg

Most people agree that the American military involvement in Vietnam was a tragedy, and as in classical drama we can learn many lessons from the suffering inflicted and undergone by the "hero." Our concern in this book is with peacemaking and the ways of establishing peace in the world. From this perspective the official policies of the United States government were a colossal failure, since U.S. influence in Vietnam resulted in the opposite of peace until the United States finally withdrew all of its influence. Even from the military point of view Indochina was the only war the U.S.A. has ever really "lost," and it happened while America was generally considered to be the greatest military power in the history of the world and at the hands of an "enemy" who was considered "primitive" and "weak." Perhaps never before has history so clearly shown the stupidity, folly, and utter ineptness of using bombing and killing to try to solve human problems. Psychologically we may come to see that those problems were more in American attitudes than in the situations of the Vietnamese except insofar as they suffered from American "influence." In this chapter we will explore how those attitudes created a terrible situation and how we can change in order to prevent such misery and failures in the future.

When World War II began, the area in Southeast Asia now known as Vietnam, Cambodia, and Laos was a colony called French Indochina. The French colonial government there declared allegiance to the Vichy regime which the Nazis established in southern France after their invasion. During that war the Japanese, as allies of the Nazis, occupied Indochina and ruled through the French colonial administration until the Vichy

211

regime in France fell. The Japanese then set up Vietnamese Emperor Bao Dai to rule over the Vietnamese. Since 1940 a guerilla resistance movement known as the Viet Minh, led by Communist Ho Chi Minh, had struggled against the Vichy French colonialists and the Japanese invaders. They were even aided by the United States and trained by their advisors. In August 1945 when the Japanese surrendered to the Allies, a popular revolution swept Vietnam and placed the Viet Minh in power. Under Ho Chi Minh's chairmanship the government of the Democratic Republic of Vietnam (DRV) was established on September 2, 1945, and the Declaration of Independence which Ho had written was announced. He quoted from the American Declaration of Independence and from the French Revolution's 1791 Declaration of Human and Civic Rights in order to appeal to the human rights principles of these two nations. As the Americans had done two centuries before, he listed the grievances the people had suffered under their colonial overlords, in this case the French. The document concludes:

> Vietnam has the right to be free and independent and, in fact, has become free and independent. The people of Vietnam decide to mobilize all their spiritual and material forces and to sacrifice their lives and property in order to safeguard their right of liberty and independence.

Although President Roosevelt had wanted to see Vietnam under a United Nations trusteeship to prepare it for independence, at the Potsdam Conference President Truman and British Prime Minister Attlee agreed to divide French Indochina at the sixteenth parallel, leaving China in control in the north and giving the British operational control over southern Vietnam. The DRV accepted this and welcomed British troops into Saigon in September. However, some dissenting Vietnamese Trotskyists were arrested and killed. The British then attacked the independence forces of the Vietnamese in order to restore to power the French colonial government in the south. The United States tacitly accepted French sovereignty over Indochina, and President Truman neglected to respond to several letters of appeal from Ho Chi Minh. Yet General

MacArthur complained, "If there is anything that makes my blood boil, it is to see our Allies in Indochina and Java deploying Japanese troops to reconquer the little people we promised to liberate. It is the most ignoble kind of betrayal."

In February 1946 France and China agreed to let French troops replace the Chinese north of the sixteenth parallel. Ho Chi Minh negotiated with the French for a free Vietnamese state within the French Union. The agreement of March called for 15,000 French troops in the north along with 10,000 Vietnamese soldiers. Ho Chi Minh and some compatriots traveled to France for a conference; the rest of the delegation soon left in protest, but Ho stayed on to bargain for a *modus vivendi* which recognized some political freedoms of the Viet Minh in the south. Returning in October 1946 Ho Chi Minh pleaded with the armies of the Vietnamese and French to stop fighting, saying, "If we use the right words, they will certainly listen to us. Violent actions are absolutely forbidden. This is what you have to do at present to create a peaceful atmosphere, paving the way democratically to reach the unification of our Vietnam." However, in November the French commander at Haiphong used a minor customs clash as a justification for launching an all-out French attack on the city. The Viet Minh were driven into the countryside, and the guerilla war against the French had begun. Not only did the United States fail to support the rights of the Vietnamese people for self-determination, but the Truman Administration gave military aid to France for its colonial war in Vietnam.

After the Chinese Communist revolution in 1949 the United States decided to increase its military aid to the French in Vietnam. In January 1950 China and the Soviet Union recognized the government of Ho Chi Minh. Dreadfully afraid of the Communists, the United States government wanted to help the French destroy the Viet Minh, but it could not publicly justify supporting a colonial war. Therefore Bao Dai, who had been in exile in Hong Kong for three years, was nominally recognized by France as the independent government of Vietnam. This enabled American military assistance to go to France while Bao Dai was the "publicized" recipient. On May 8, 1950 Secretary of State Dean Acheson made the following statement:

The United States Government, convinced that neither national independence nor democratic evolution exist in any area dominated by Soviet imperialism, considers the situation to be such as to warrant its according economic aid and military equipment to the Associated States of Indochina and to France in order to assist them in restoring stability and permitting these states to pursue their peaceful and democratic development.

To compare objectively this attitude to the facts of the situation, one cannot help but see the American paranoia and hypocrisy. First, America was helping France to squelch Vietnamese national independence and democratic evolution with imperialistic war and colonial oppression. Second, the only Soviet involvement was a simple diplomatic statement toward a purely ideological ally. Even aid from the Chinese Communists was minimal during this period. Yet from 1950 to 1954 the United States gave the Bao Dai government $126 million in economic, military, and technical assistance while supplying the French with $2.6 billion of military material, which accounted for four-fifths of the French military effort. With Eisenhower's election in 1952 the new Secretary of State, John Foster Dulles, expressed the paranoia as the "Domino Theory." The Korean War was fought for these same reasons during this period.

In spite of the military power of France aided by the United States the Viet Minh were able to win an impressive victory at Dienbienphu in 1954. The French were ready now to give up control of Vietnam, and they agreed to an armistice at Geneva. However, the document was never signed by any of the parties, because the United States refused to give even its oral consent. U.S. officials wanted France to continue the struggle. Although President Eisenhower considered using tactical nuclear weapons or sending U.S. troops, he had the good sense not to involve America in another land war in Asia. Dulles tried to consolidate interests in the area with the Southeast Asia Treaty Organization (SEATO), but only Thailand, Pakistan, and the Philippines agreed to assist each other against outside aggression.

The Geneva accords removed the French from northern Vietnam and recognized the Bao Dai government in the south for the two years the French had been given to depart from there. Then an election was supposed to unify the country. This temporary concession of southern territory by the Vietnamese to the French was a response to strong pressure from the Soviet and Chinese representatives Molotov and Chou En-Lai. The French left on schedule but were replaced in May 1955 by the United States and its military support for South Vietnam. Bao Dai was replaced by the pro-American dictator, Ngo Dinh Diem, who refused to hold elections because the Communists would have won. Diem re-established the landlords who had been removed by guerillas for supporting the Japanese and the French. The peasants of the Viet Minh rebelled, and guerilla fighting spread. Diem violated every article of the constitution and had thousands of people imprisoned in camps. By 1959 United States military "advisors" were being killed in Vietnam, and in 1960 the guerillas formed the National Liberation Front (NLF). The Second Indochina War had begun.

Most of the NLF were southern Vietnamese. Very few northern troops entered South Vietnam until the American troops had arrived in force. The Americans were attempting to hold back a revolution more than prevent an invasion; it was primarily a civil war. On December 20, 1960 the National Liberation Front formulated the following Ten Points:

1) Overthrow the camouflaged colonial regime of the American imperialists and the dictatorial power of Ngo Dinh Diem, servant of the Americans, and institute a government of national democratic union.
2) Institute a largely liberal and democratic regime.
3) Establish an independent and sovereign economy, and improve the living conditions of the people.
4) Reduce land rent; implement agrarian reform with the aim of providing land to the tillers.
5) Develop a national and democratic culture and education.

6) Create a national army devoted to the defense of the Fatherland and the people.

7) Guarantee equality between the various minorities and between the sexes; protect the legitimate interests of foreign citizens established in Vietnam and of Vietnamese citizens residing abroad.

8) Promote a foreign policy of peace and neutrality.

9) Re-establish normal relations between the two zones, and prepare for the peaceful reunification of the country.

10) Struggle against all aggressive war; actively defend universal peace.

In the full manifesto each of these points was followed by several specific means of implementation. For example, point 2 included the following: abolishing the dictatorial powers of Diem and electing a National Assembly through universal suffrage; implementing essential democratic liberties such as freedom of opinion, press, assembly, movement, trade-unionism, religion, and political organizations; proclaiming a general amnesty for all political prisoners and abolishing fascist and antidemocratic laws; and prohibiting all illegal arrests, detentions, and torture. The Twelve Points of Discipline for the People's Liberation Army suggested the following conduct for soldiers toward civilians: "Be fair and honest in business with the people . . . Never take even a needle from the people . . . When staying in civilian houses, maintain it as if it is one's own . . . Be polite with the people and love the people." With these ideals as standards, it is no wonder that the NLF made such successful inroads in South Vietnam!

By 1961 more than half of South Vietnamese territory was under Communist control. Over the next two years President Kennedy sent sixteen thousand American soldiers as advisors to the South Vietnamese army. In May 1963 the Buddhists rebelled against Diem's tyrannical government, and monks began setting themselves on fire in protest. The United States hinted that changes in the government were needed. On November 1 a military coup deposed Diem, and he and his brother Nhu were assassinated. Over the next year and a half the government of

South Vietnam changed hands among the Generals several times. In February 1964 President Lyndon Johnson issued public warnings to North Vietnam and ordered the covert bombing of Laos near the border of North Vietnam. In Augrust the *U.S.S. Maddox* was attacked while patrolling in the Gulf of Tonkin, probably in retaliation for a South Vietnamese Navy attack on an island in the north two days before. The *Maddox* fired back, and two days later another attack was reported. The U.S. ships were not damaged nor were any Americans hurt, while they had sunk three or four of the attacking torpedo boats. Nevertheless Johnson ordered sixty-four bombing sorties over four North Vietnamese bases, and he requested approval from Congress to use armed forced. This excessive response has been considered a violation of the rules of civilized warfare as interpreted in the Nuremberg trials. Senator Wayne Morse declared that the Gulf of Tonkin Resolution gave the President "war-making powers in the absence of a declaration of war," and he lamented that it was a historic mistake.

On February 7, 1965 President Johnson, who had been overwhelmingly elected over Goldwater's militaristic and reactionary programs, ordered the bombing of North Vietnam. The next day the Students for a Democratic Society (SDS) issued a statement of outrage, saying that the U.S. was supporting dictatorship, not freedom, and was intervening in a civil war, not a war of aggression. SDS asked, "What kind of America is it whose response to poverty and oppression in Vietnam is napalm and defoliation? . . . How many more lives must be lost before the Johnson Administration accepts the foregone conclusions?" A graduated bombing program was begun in March, and in April the United States began sending thousands of combat troops to South Vietnam.

Also in April Hanoi offered its proposal for a settlement consisting of four points in accordance with the 1954 Geneva agreements: 1) recognition of Vietnamese independence and territorial integrity by withdrawal of all U.S. forces, bases, and weapons; 2) no foreign military bases or troops in Vietnam and no military alliances for the two zones; 3) settlement of South Vietnamese affairs according to the program of the NLF; and 4)

217

peaceful reunification of Vietnam without any foreign interference. This proposal was rejected in Washington out of hand, because they assumed the NLF program would exclude other groups. During Thanksgiving weekend there was a peace march in Washington, and the anti-war leaders urged the Communists to respond to American peace initiatives. Ho Chi Minh replied that the four points still held, and that the U.S. must ease its criminal war of aggression against Vietnam. At Christmas the U.S. temporarily halted the bombing, hoping for some capitulation from North Vietnam. Hanoi replied that the United States was thousands of miles away and had no right to invade South Vietnam or to impose conditions on the DRV. On December 21, 1965 the United Nations passed a resolution declaring that no state has the right to intervene in the affairs of another state and condemning armed intervention. It declared, "Every state has an inalienable right to choose its political, economic, social and cultural systems, without interference in any form by another state." A Citizens' White Paper by Schurmann, Scott, and Zelnik studying nine critical periods from November 1963 to July 1966 concluded, "Movements toward a political settlement have been retarded or broken off by American interventions, most of which have taken the form of military escalation."

By 1967 nearly half a million American soldiers were fighting in South Vietnam. In November General Westmoreland announced that troop withdrawal could begin in 1969 if the bombing and military progress continued. However, on the Vietnamese holiday of Tet at the end of January 1968 the Viet Cong (NLF) launched a massive attack on the major cities of South Vietnam. Within three weeks about 165,000 civilians had been killed, and there were two million new refugees. An American major looking at the devastated village of Ben Tre, said, "We had to destroy it in order to save it." The offensive, which included an invasion of the U.S. Embassy in Saigon, came as a great shock to Americans. The huge size of the action and its surprise to the Americans and South Vietnamese Army indicated that most of the people in the country were more loyal to the NLF than to the government.

When Westmoreland and Chief of Staff General Wheeler asked for 200,000 more troops, President Johnson was visibly shaken and began to doubt seriously for the first time the military policies he was following. In March Senator Eugene McCarthy won a victory in the New Hampshire Presidential primary running against Johnson's Vietnam war policy. A few days later Robert Kennedy announced his candidacy. On March 31 President Johnson announced he would not seek re-election, and to begin de-escalation of the war he limited the bombing to a small strategic area. The war and the anti-war movement that had been aroused to protest it had ruined the Johnson Presidency, which on domestic issues had been rather successful. In May formal negotiations began in Paris, but with the election of Richard Nixon, American involvement in Indochina was to drag on for five more years.

The peace movement continued to grow and affected Nixon's policies as well. President Nixon wanted to strike a "savage blow" against North Vietnam in the fall of 1969 by mining Haiphong harbor and perhaps even using nuclear weapons, but the demonstrations were so large in October and November that he changed his mind for political reasons. For example, on November 9 a full-page ad appeared in the *New York Times* signed by 1365 active duty GI's, saying, "We are opposed to American involvement in the war in Vietnam. We resent the needless wasting of lives to save face for the politicians in Washington." The story of the massacre of over seven hundred civilians at My Lai was exposed to public outcry. On November 15 three quarters of a million people gathered in Washington while one quarter of a million marched in San Francisco.

When Nixon ordered the invasion of Cambodia in May 1970, strikes on American college campuses involved over four million students. In June the Senate repealed the Gulf of Tonkin Resolution and barred future U.S. military operations in Cambodia without Congressional approval. Adapting to public pressure, President Nixon began withdrawing U.S. troops, but he kept the war going by bombing Laos, Cambodia, and North Vietnam. The "Vietnamization" of the war was doomed to fail without U.S. support. Running against the peace candidate

McGovern in 1972 Nixon promised peace, and a cease-fire agreement was signed in January 1973. However, it was only when the Watergate scandal began to weaken the Nixon Presidency that Congress, on July 1, 1973, finally cut off all funds for any military activity in Indochina.

What were the results of American military involvement in Vietnam? Without American support the government of South Vietnam completely collapsed by 1975. More than three million Americans were sent to Vietnam. Nearly 58,000 were killed, and about 300,000 were wounded. A conservative estimate of *civilian* casualties in South Vietnam was the Senate Subcommittee on Refugees estimates of 400,000 killed, 900,000 wounded, and 6.4 million turned into refugees. The United States dropped from the air 3.2 million tons of bombs on South Vietnam, 2.1 million tons on Laos (almost one ton per person), and 340,000 tons on North Vietnam. Both Johnson and Nixon each presided over more bombing than all of World War II. An obvious result of American military involvement is that the people of Vietnam were terribly militarized for self-defense and forced to try to solve their problems with military means. The legacy of this goes on.

In South Vietnam alone the United States government directly spent $141 billion. In other words, in a country where the per capita income is $157 per year, the U.S. poured in the equivalent of $7,000 per person for the twenty million inhabitants. Most of this was spent destructively, but another result was the most decadent type of economy involving large amounts of graft, favoritism, prostitution, and drugs. The world's most powerful and wealthy nation was unable to defeat an army of peasants using homemade and captured weapons. Ostensibly fighting to preserve freedom the United States propped up a series of military dictators. The American forces traveled halfway around the world to attack Vietnamese people in North and South Vietnam supposedly to protect them from "external agression." The only conceivable external aggression, other than that of the U.S., was the movement of people from North Vietnam to South Vietnam; yet the basis of the Geneva Accords was that Vietnam was to be one country. Then how can the movement of Vietnamese in their own country be considered external aggression? The United States claimed it must continue the fight for its honor and the respect of its allies; yet never before has America been so dishonored or lost the respect of its allies more than it did in Vietnam.

Using the weak justification of SEATO's collective defense arrangements the United States violated the United Nations Charter, the Geneva Accords of 1954, the Nuremberg Code, the Hague Convention, the Geneva Protocol of 1925, and the Paris agreements of 1973. Legal expert Richard A. Falk noted the following illegal war policies: "1) the Phoenix Program, 2) aerial and naval bombardment of undefended villages, 3) destruction of crops and forests, 4) 'search-and-destroy' missions, 5) 'harassment and interdiction' fire, 6) forcible removal of civilian population, 7) reliance on a variety of weapons prohibited by treaty." After devastating the country of Vietnam, the United States has not even considered paying reparations. In fact the U.S. was the only nation out of 141 that refused to endorse a United Nations resolution urging priority economic assistance to Vietnam.

Another result is the terrible injuries, both physical and psychological, which the Vietnam veterans must learn to live with. The moral problems have caused severe psychological disturbances. Hundreds of thousands of Americans were trained to kill and did kill hundreds of thousands of Vietnamese. When they discovered it was for no good reason, the remorse, grief, guilt, anger, frustration, and resentment erupted. The number of veterans who have committed suicide is larger than the number of Americans killed in Vietnam. The veterans bear the heaviest psychological burden, but all Americans are responsible.

The only restraints on U.S. military escalation were the fear of a conflict with China or the Soviet Union and the conscience of the American public as represented in the peace movement. Noting that anti-war demonstrators did not kill a single person during the period the U.S. government killed hundreds of thousands in Indochina, Fred Halstead summarized the accomplishments of the anti-war movement as breaking the spell of anticommunist hysteria, increasing healthy skepticism of political leaders, changing the stereotype of soldiers as obedient pawns, becoming reluctant to engage in military adventures abroad, and expanding social reform movements to issues of foreign policy. For the first time in American history the people successfully challenged the government's right to wage war.

Why, then, did America get bogged down in the quagmire of Vietnam for so long at such great cost? After World War II the United States became the greatest power in the history of the world. The abuse of greatness is the abuse of the power. America thought it could do no wrong. At the same time Americans had a tremendous fear of Communism. Historically, it took a decade and a half before the U.S. even recognized the Soviet Union and more than two decades before it recognized nearly a billion people in China. With a world-wide military force the United States was arrogant enough to think that it could stop Communism by force of arms. Psychologically there was the irrational fear that if America did not intervene, somehow Communism would take over the world. The Soviet empire was likewise afraid of encroachment through Korea or eastern Europe and therefore took steps to place a protective ring around itself, while the United States has protective military bases all around the world.

Because of this combination of American power, fear of Communism, and self-righteous concepts about democracy, the U.S. foolishly tried to set up a non-Communist government in a country that was trying to free itself from French colonialism by a combination of nationalistic independence and Communist ideology. Only by the influence of its military power could the United States try to hold back the tide of political revolution and true national independence in Vietnam.

What are the lessons for the future the United States can learn? Military methods ultimately do not solve political and social problems. True independence and self-determination are best attained without military interference. Military methods only militarize the opposition and escalate violence so that peaceful solutions are more unattainable. The security of the United States and its allies is not really threatened by what goes on in small underdeveloped countries. Nuclear weapons are of no use in these situations. Armed intervention will eventually backfire.

The U.S. has no legal right to be a policeman in another country. The veterans can teach others of the horrors and agonies of war. The American people must not allow the President to go astray while intoxicated with power. An effective peace movement can dramatically influence political policies. Finally, every person has the responsibility to refuse to support an illegal and immoral war.

21
The Clark-Sohn Proposal for World Law and Disarmament

"What can fairly be called peace
is the result only of enforceable law;
under modern conditions,
general disarmament is the precondition
of enforceable world law."

Grenville Clark

"The proposition 'no peace without law'
also embodies the conception that
peace cannot be ensured by a continued arms race,
nor by an indefinite 'balance of terror,'
nor by diplomatic maneuver,
but only by universal and complete national disarmament
together with the establishment of institutions
corresponding in the world field to those which
maintain law and order within local communities and nations."

Clark and Sohn

"Either world problems will be settled
through real world organization, meaning world law,
or they will be settled by world war."

Norman Cousins

Many philosophers and proponents of world peace have expressed ideas similar to the credo of the World Federalists, that world peace depends upon world justice which depends upon enforceable world law which depends upon world government. The most discussed plan for effective world law is the comprehensive proposal to strengthen the United Nations delineated by Grenville Clark and Louis B. Sohn in their book *World Peace Through World Law.*

Grenville Clark graduated from Harvard Law School in 1906. Foreseeing the likelihood of American involvement in the first world war, he put forward the "Plattsburgh Idea" which led to the recruitment of 60,000 line officers between 1915 and 1917. During the war he served in the United States Army. At the beginning of World War II when the Nazis had occupied

Norway, he initiated the Selective Service Act of 1940 to prepare the U.S. for the war. He served as a consultant to Secretary of War Stimson for the next four years.

Turning his attention to the prevention of war, Clark published *A Plan for Peace* in 1950. In this book Clark asserts that disarmament supported by "institutions of world law through a world federation of universal membership" is the only real hope for enduring peace. He recommends a federal structure in which all powers not expressly delegated to war prevention be reserved to the nations and their peoples. In the promotion of economic and social welfare the powers of United Nations agencies to *inquire* and *recommend* should be strengthened. Written from an American perspective, Clark's plan was submitted to the United States Congress. Five essential points of the plan are to: 1) encourage discussion of the shocking implications of a third world war; 2) recognize that complete disarmament is necessary to a stable and peaceful world, and that disarmament requires effective world law and government; 3) urge the United States to explore proposals for disarmament and revision of the United Nations; 4) maintain military resistance to Communist expansion while working toward an overall settlement; and 5) realize that executive officials need new ideas from the people and help from Congress.

Clark explains why the "peace by strength" doctrine of deterrence is so insecure and leads to a continuous arms race. In deterring Russia the United States has also alarmed her, resulting in a vicious circle in which each side accuses the other of aggression and imperialism, while each increases its armaments, engendering more suspicion and fear, and thus more armaments, etc. A Pax Americana achieved through conquest, like the Pax Romana, can never last. A constructive plan for general disarmament and enforceable world law is needed.

Clark faces the obstacles to his plan and also looks at the counterforces working in its favor. The nations' reluctance to modify their claims to unlimited sovereignty is a major problem. People must overcome their fear of "foreigners" and develop a world consciousness. Conflicts of religion, particularly between Christians and Communists, could be a stumbling block, but with some tolerance it should not prevent a solution. Recriminations between the East and West are a great psychological handicap, but this atmosphere can be improved with effort. Pessimism that such a new system could ever be instituted in a short time can be a negative, self-fulfilling prophecy, but again, working for a realistic solution can dissolve that attitude. Skepticism about the Russians' willingness to negotiate in reasonable terms is a common attitude in America. Yet a plan that is in everyone's interest would be beneficial to Russians as well as Americans.

Most of the counterforces to these obstacles are steadily increasing in strength. The severity of modern war is becoming worse rapidly. A world war is becoming more likely to be instant mass suicide. Self-interest is enhanced with world order. The crushing economic burden of armaments would be drastically reduced, and the psychological relief could be euphoric. Besides the problem of the super-power rivalry, there is a general need for peace to prevent the various small wars and to use resources to improve the general welfare. The federal principle of government is being understood by more people because of political evolution in various countries and regions. New generations are producing new leaders with new ideas that are more appropriate to our new problems. Clark had great vision, and he prophetically remarked that a crisis often gets worse until the proud opponents look down into the dark abyss that awaits them if they do not change. The closer we get to the brink of disaster, the more likely we are to find a solution.

Louis B. Sohn was born in Lwow, Poland the year World War I began. He earned his first law degree at John Casimir University in Lwow. He participated in the San Francisco Conference that established the United Nations, and he was a legal officer in the United Nations Secretariat for two years. Since 1951 he has been on the faculty at Harvard Law School. In recent years he has been working on the Law of the Sea Treaty.

Clark and Sohn collaborated in suggesting a Revised United Nations Charter in their book *World Peace Through World Law,* which was first published in 1958. They refined their ideas in a second, revised edition in 1960. Subsequent revisions in 1966 and

1973 offered an additional alternative to a revised UN Charter by suggesting a new world security and development organization to supplement current UN functions. This discussion will focus on the proposed UN Charter Revision.

The basic premise agrees with President Eisenhower's statement in 1956, "There can be no peace without law." Thus for world peace, enforceable world law is required. By presenting a detailed plan Clark and Sohn hope to stimulate world-wide discussion of the needed world institutions. World law is essential because of the increasing number and destructive power of modern weapons, because more nations are acquiring nuclear weapons, and because of the resources wasted on the arms race; in 1973 Sohn added the concern about protecting the environment and natural resources. They proposed revising the United Nations, because of the UN's established functions and purpose of preventing war. However, they admit that forming a new institution could also serve the same principles. In fact, in 1962 Clark and Sohn formulated their proposals in the form of a comprehensive Draft Treaty between the U.S. and U.S.S.R., which would not require revision of the UN Charter.

The Clark-Sohn Plan is based on these principles. First, genuine peace depends on an effective system of world law which can ensure complete disarmament by means of institutions to clearly state the law, courts to apply the law, and police to enforce the law. Second, world law must be formulated in a constitution and statutes forbidding nations to use violence, except in self-defense, and must be applicable to all nations and individuals. Third, world judicial tribunals and organs of mediation and conciliation must be established in order to use peaceful means of adjudication instead of violence or the threat of violence in the solving of all international disputes. Fourth, a permanent world police force must be maintained, with careful safeguards against abuse, in order to "suppress any violation of the world law against international violence." Fifth, complete disarmament of all nations must be "accomplished in a simultaneous and proportionate manner by carefully verified stages subject to a well-organized system of inspection." Sixth, the tremendous disparities in the economic conditions of different regions of the world must be lessened by world institutions in order to resolve conflicts and instability. Seventh, humanity's common resources and environment must be managed and protected equitably. Supplementary principles suggest that the world law must apply to all nations and individuals, and nearly all nations must be actively participating in the institutions. Also, the basic rights and duties of all nations should be clearly defined in the constitutional document with the world body's powers limited primarily to the area of war prevention, while all other powers are reserved to the nations and their peoples.

Now let us briefly outline the features of the Clark-Sohn Plan for a Revised Charter of the United Nations. For the plan to go into effect, nearly every major nation must agree to become a member. Every independent state in the world would be eligible for membership, and ratification would require at least five-sixths of all nations, nations combining at least five-sixths of the world population, plus all four of the largest nations and at least six of the ten next largest nations in population. The few remaining non-member nations would be required to comply with the disarmament plan and world law.

Voting in the General Assembly would be adjusted according to a nation's population, and the Assembly would be given adequate powers to maintain peace and enforce the disarmament process. The 1973 Clark-Sohn voting proposal suggests the following: the four largest nations would have 30 representatives each; the next ten largest nations would have 12 each; the next fifteen nations would have 8 each; the next twenty nations 6 each; the next thirty nations 4 each; the next forty nations 3 each; and the smallest nations, those with under one million inhabitants, would have one representative each. This particular scheme of weighted voting is perhaps one of the weakest elements of their plan, but they admit that they are not dogmatic about its specifics. Certainly, if the General Assembly is going to be given greater powers, some system which takes into account the population differences among nations must be devised. Clark and Sohn suggest stages eventually leading to the election of representatives by popular vote, although at first some nations would probably insist on choosing them in their national legislatures.

An Executive Council would replace the Security Council, and the veto power would be abolished. The four largest nations (China, India, U.S., and U.S.S.R.) would be permanent members. Five of the ten largest nations would alternate with the other five as members, and the remaining eight members would be chosen by the Assembly. "Important" matters would require a vote of twelve of the seventeen members, a majority of the nine larger nations, and a majority of the eight other members. The Economic and Social Council and the Trusteeship Council would be continued and enlarged for greater responsibilities subject to the General Assembly.

Disarmament is carefully worked out by Clark and Sohn to eliminate national military forces in a step-by-step process. Complete disarmament down to the level of local police is required because of the destructive power of modern weapons. Even a small number of nuclear weapons or biological and chemical weapons would leave the world very insecure, and they would make it difficult for the world police force to deter or suppress international violence. Besides, nations would not need armies if the world police force is protecting every nation and their people from international aggression. Each nation would need only enough police forces and weapons to quell internal disruptions and the violence of criminals.

The original Clark-Sohn Plan schedules the verified disarmament process over twelve years, but the Draft Treaty cuts that time in half. Nevertheless, the process is essentially the same. The first two years (or one in the Draft Treaty) would stop further military build-up, establish the UN Inspection Service to make a detailed arms census for every nation, and allow time to verify those facts. Then each nation would disarm ten percent of their forces each year (or six months) for the next ten years (or five years). Each step would be carefully verified by the Inspection Service, and if necessary the process would be delayed until compliance was achieved. A Nuclear Energy Authority would become responsible for all nuclear materials. An Outer Space Agency would also be created to ensure the peaceful use of space. Some of the national armaments would be given to the UN Peace Force, which would come up to its full strength by the end of the disarmament process. Every nation in the world would be bound by the disarmament and at its conclusion would be reduced to lightly armed police.

A World Police Force would be the only military force permitted in the world, once disarmament was completed. Clark and Sohn have devised various safeguards to prevent any nation from taking control of the World Force. Thus major roles are given to people from the smaller countries. This force would be under the direction of the General Assembly and would have between 200,000 and 400,000 professional soldiers, drawn mostly from the smaller nations. No more than three percent of the force could be nationals from any one nation, and the forces would be scattered around the globe in various regions with no permanent military bases in any of the larger countries. A Peace Force Reserve would have between 300,000 and 600,000 volunteers on call in case of an emergency. The Peace Force would be equipped with the most modern weapons, but biological, chemical, and nuclear weapons would be forbidden. If nuclear weapons somehow were illegally produced and became a threat, the General Assembly could order the Nuclear Energy Authority to release nuclear weapons to the Peace Force. Otherwise nuclear weapons would be forever banned. A Military Staff Committee of five persons drawn from the smaller nations would direct the Peace Force under the civilian authority of the Executive Council and ultimately the General Assembly.

The Revised Charter requires every nation to settle all international disputes by peaceful means such as "negotiation, enquiry, mediation, conciliation, arbitration, judicial settlement," etc. All nations would be obligated to submit any "legal question," which in the opinion of the General Assembly (or the Executive Council) endangers the peace of the world, to the International Court of Justice for a final and binding decision. Those disputes which are not of a legal nature would be brought to the World Conciliation Board for a voluntary agreement or would be referred to the World Equity Tribunal for a solution which could be made binding by the General Assembly. The International Court of Justice would have compulsory jurisdiction on all cases submitted to it by the

Assembly as well as disputes over treaties, international agreements, and the UN Charter. Individuals responsible for violations of the disarmament provisions could also be prosecuted. A civil police force of less than 10,000 would aid the Inspection Service in detecting such violators.

A World Development Authority would aid the underdeveloped areas of the world in improving their economic conditions in order to alleviate the immense disparities between their circumstances and those of the industrialized nations. A United Nations Ocean Authority would manage the resources of the seas. A UN Environmental Protection Authority would coordinate environmental programs, collect data, and monitor and assess services. As of 1973 Sohn suggests $75 billion for world development, $12 billion for the Peace Forces, and $3 billion for the other agencies. This budget of $90 billion represents less than half of the world's military expeditures for the year 1970. Obviously the world economy would be greatly enhanced by such a plan. They also suggest an over-all limit of three percent of the gross world product for the UN budget. Each nation would be taxed by the General Assembly according to its gross national product with a "per capita deduction" for the poorest nations. No nation could be taxed more than four percent of its GNP, and each nation would collect its own taxes for the UN fiscal office in the nation. Once the Revised UN Charter was ratified, no nation would be allowed to withdraw.

A Bill of Rights is annexed to the Revised Charter to protect individual rights such as freedom of religion, communication, assembly and petition, and a fair trial without double jeopardy, *ex post facto* laws, excessive bail, cruel and unusual punishments, unlawful detention, and unreasonable searches and seizures. The many useful organs of the UN would be continued, such as the Food and Agriculture Organization (FAO), the United Nations Educational, Scientific and Cultural Organization (UNESCO), the International Labor Organization (ILO), and the World Health Organization (WHO). The purpose of the Clark-Sohn Plan is not to delete any of these useful functions but to strengthen the UN's ability to prevent war by making the General Assembly and Security Council more representative and filling the major lacks of the UN, namely the lack of effective disarmament, the lack of a standing world police force, the lack of a judicial system with compulsory jurisdiction over international disputes, and the lack of a reliable revenue system.

To the obstacles Clark saw in 1950, Sohn adds the resistance of the vested interests in armament, both in the military and industry, as well as the vested interests in traditional diplomacy. However, the advanced "delivery systems" of nuclear weapons have made the problem much more urgent. In addition, pollution of the environment is becoming more critical as is the disparity between the developed Northern hemisphere and the underdeveloped Southern hemisphere.

The year after the Clark-Sohn Plan was first proposed, Soviet Premier Khrushchev visited the United Nations and on September 19, 1959 suggested in a speech that general and complete disarmament could be the best approach to peace. The United States, among others, responded favorably to the idea. Two years and six days later U.S. President Kennedy told the UN General Assembly, "To destroy arms, however, is not enough. We must create even as we destroy — creating world-wide law and law enforcement as we outlaw world-wide war and weapons." He suggested that UN machinery be improved to provide for "the peaceful settlement of disputes, for on-the-spot factfinding, mediation and adjudication, for extending the rule of international law." On September 20, 1961 the Soviet Union and the United States issued a "Joint Statement of Agreed Principles for Disarmament Negotiations" known as the McCloy-Zorin Agreement. This agreement declares, "The programme for general and complete disarmament shall ensure that States will have at their disposal only such non-nuclear armaments, forces, facilities and establishments as are agreed to be necessary to maintaining internal order and protect the personal security of citizens; and that States shall support and provide agreed manpower for a United Nations peace force," and it calls for the disbanding of all military establishments, "the elimination of all stockpiles of nuclear, chemical, bacteriological and other weapons of mass destruction" and their delivery systems, and "the discontinuance of military expenditures." It suggests that disarmament be implemented in stages with adequate verification for each stage by effective international control. It recommends "the widest possible agreement at the earliest possible date."

In the first half of 1962 both the Soviet Union and the United States put forward draft treaties for general and complete disarmament. In May 1962 Clark and Sohn recast their proposals as a "Proposed Treaty Establishing a World Disarmament and World Development Organization within the Framework of the United Nations." The U.S. proposal would give the International Court jurisdiction over diputes on the disarmament during the first stage, while the Soviet version does not mention the International Court at all. The Clark-Sohn Plan offers incentives to most people in the world with its development provisions, but the Soviet and U.S. proposals ignore this need. The Soviets were reluctant to give up their veto in the Security Council, and the American proposal is vague on how the UN would enforce disarmament. However, the Clark-Sohn treaty would give the new disarmament organization enforcement authority. The Soviet Treaty would lead to a disarmed world, but it would not provide a workable system for settling international disputes. The U.S. treaty would begin to try to deal with international conflicts only after the first stage of disarmement. Both the U.S. and Soviet plans would result in a balance of national power instead of the world-based enforceable world law of the Clark-Sohn approach. The Clark-Sohn Plan has the advantage of solving unanswered questions prior to agreement and implementation so that confidence in the future can be gained. Obviously none of these proposals have been implemented. After the Cuban missile crisis in October 1962 the Soviets decided to catch up with the U.S. in the nuclear arms race.

The Clark-Sohn proposals were presented as a useful basis for discussion of these questions, and they have in fact stimulated a great deal of thought. Saul Mendlovitz and Richard Falk used *World Peace Through World Law* as a foundation upon which to build elaborate teaching materials for discussions on world order. The Institute for World Order is still developing outstanding educational materials from experts around the world in their World Order Models Project (WOMP). Such notables as Herman Kahn and Andrei Sakharov have recommended careful study of the Clark-Sohn proposals. As early as 1973 these materials had been studied in about 500 colleges and universities in the United States.

Why have these ideas not yet succeeded? Richard Falk points out in a *Study of Future Worlds* that change-oriented groups have not been responsive to law-based appeals, which are at the same time both radical and conservative. Law and order is a conservative approach, while giving up national sovereignty to world institutions is a radical change. Amitai Etzioni in *The Hard Way to Peace* asks what can be done to accelerate the historical processes that will lead to these solutions. He suggests the formation of supranational communities and also economic and political development around the world. As Falk and Mendlovitz have concisely summarized, the Clark-Sohn Plan provides "an international legal framework within which the widest possible shaping and sharing of the values of human dignity can take place."

22
Women and Peace

*"If nonviolence is the law of our being,
the future is with women."*

Mahatma Gandhi

*"Our function is to establish new values,
to create an overpowering sense of the sacredness of life,
so that war will be unthinkable;
so that when international disputes arise,
even of the most grave character — when lives have been lost,
when our rights have been clearly invaded —
we shall not turn to wholesale, deliberate destruction of life
as the means of settling those disputes,
of avenging those deaths, of asserting those rights."*

Crystal Eastman

*"As women entered into politics
when clean milk and premature labor of children
became factors in political life,
so they might be concerned with international affairs
when these at least were dealing with
such human and poignant matters as food for starving peoples
who could be fed only through international activities . . .
There might be found an antidote to war in woman's affection
and all-embracing pity for helpless children."*

Jane Addams

"Love is the measure by which we will be judged."

Dorothy Day

*"Feminism can help women respect their own power.
Nonviolence can help them use their power effectively
in a way which maintains that respect
and extends it to others."*

Jane Meyerding

"Experiment with nonviolent struggle has barely begun.
But in a world in which traditional violent battle
can escalate into nuclear war,
it is an experiment that is absolutely necessary
to push to its furthest limits."

Barbara Deming

This chapter is probably as important as all of the previous chapters combined, for women make up more than half of the human race. Civilization has been suffering for more than four thousand years under the aggressive oppression of male dominance and authoritarian patriarchy. Some of the great philosophers of peace, such as 'Abdu'l-Baha and Gandhi, have seen hope for a peaceful world in the future because of the softening of masculine force by the feminine qualities of love, service, intuition, and moral power. The women's movement is well on the way to healing a society so afflicted by militarism that it teeters on the brink of mass destruction. Whereas war used to be a masculine "sport" for warriors, in the twentieth century the percentage of civilian deaths in war has steadily increased until now everyone is imperiled by the threat of nuclear holocaust. At the same time women have become increasingly involved in actively working for peace, responding instinctively to nurture the human race for the sake of its survival.

In the late sixteenth century six Indian tribes were confederated into the Iroquois League for the sake of peace. Nevertheless the warriors' desire for individual glory led to much fighting. On at least one occasion the women organized a non-cooperation campaign to stop a war in the same way that Aristophanes had dramatized it in his play *Lysistrata*.

Many people came to America for reasons of conscience and religious liberty, such as Roger Williams and later the pacifist Society of Friends. In Boston Ann Hutchinson spoke so persuasively about conscience and inner spiritual guidance that she was brought to trial and banished from Massachusetts. In 1657 this colony outlawed the Society of Friends. Several Friends disobeyed the law and taught about the "Inner Light" in Massachusetts. Three of them were hanged for this "crime," including Mary Dyer.

Prior to the American Civil War many women were leaders in efforts to abolish slavery and attain women's rights. The New England Non-Resistance Society formed in 1838 included Lucretia Mott, Sarah and Angelina Grimke, Lydia Maria Child, Maria Chapman, Abby Kelly, and Ann Weston.

Lucretia Mott was the mother of six and a strong Quaker. She criticized conservative attitudes in the Religious Society of Friends and advocated not using the products of slavery. When in 1833 William Lloyd Garrison organized the all-male American Antislavery Society in Philadelphia, Lucretia organized the Philadelphia Female Antislavery Society four days later. Angelina and Sarah Grimke joined; as they began to address "mixed" audiences, the "woman question" arose. The controversy erupted at the First Annual Convention of Antislavery Women on May 17, 1838 when a mob, angry that black and white women were meeting together before a "promiscuous" audience of men and women, burned the new Pennsylvania Hall to the ground with the apparent approval of the mayor and the police. From there the mob went to attack the Motts' home, but someone led them in the wrong direction. Lucretia Mott had led the evacuation of the hall, suggesting that the women link arms in pairs of one white woman and one black woman. She calmly awaited the mob at her home with her husband and their guests. The next day the women met again and decided to increase their efforts. At the following year's convention Lucretia refused police protection and ignored advice to keep the races apart on the streets. A few months later, her bravery prevented an abolitionist friend from being tarred and feathered in Delaware. She declared, "Take me, since I am the chief offender. I ask no favor for my sex."

In 1840 Lucretia Mott went to London for the World Antislavery Convention; even though she represented two organizations, she was not admitted. However, she met Elizabeth Cady Stanton, and in 1848 they organized the Seneca Falls Convention for women's rights. Lucretia Mott spoke always for the equal and balanced empowerment of women and men harmoniously blended so that "there would be less war, injustice, and intolerance in the world than now." She remained an active

Non-Resistant and pacifist even during the Civil War, supporting conscientious objectors and recommending only moral force.

Abby Kelly had an equal partnership with her husband, Stephen S. Foster; they alternated going on speaking tours and taking care of their child and the farm. Once when they were both arrested in Ohio for handing out antislavery literature on the Sabbath, Abby refused to cooperate and was carried to jail. After the Civil War they refused to pay taxes on their farm because women were not represented in government.

Civil disobedience was used by Susan B. Anthony and fifteen other women when they voted illegally in the election of 1872. The National Woman's Suffrage Association, led by Anthony, encouraged tax refusal and public demonstrations as well as civil disobedience.

In England the suffragist movement was led by the militant Pankhurst family, using increasingly violent methods, such as burning buildings and planting bombs. However, those in the non-militant National Union of Women's Suffrage Societies believed that nonviolent political pressure was a better method than falling into the "might is right" tactics of either side. When the world war broke out, most of the militants supported the war. Then many of the non-militants saw even more clearly how society was based on force. They decided that the work for women's rights was inseparable from peace. Many of these women joined Jane Addams at The Hague in 1915 to work for peace and international order.

Alice Paul managed to extract a militant but nonviolent approach from the Pankhursts' methods and taught it to Americans when she returned from England in 1910. She formed the Congressional Union for Woman Suffrage in 1913 and was chairperson until 1917 when it merged with the Woman's Party to become the National Woman's Party. In January of that year she began the first major demonstration in front of the White House to demand that President Wilson keep his promise to work for a woman suffrage amendment to the U.S. Constitution. The vigil continued until May 22 when the police arrested 218 women. The 97 imprisoned demanded to be treated as political prisoners, refusing to work and going on a hunger strike. In 1923

Alice Paul, who had three law degrees, wrote the first women's equal rights amendment to be introduced to Congress. In 1938 she founded the World Women's Party for Equal Rights which was able to get equal rights for women included in the United Nations Charter.

Jane Addams was born on September 6, 1860 in Cedarville, Illinois. Her mother died before she was three, and she was raised by her father, who believed in Quaker principles and served eight terms in the Illinois Senate. Illness interrupted Jane's medical studies. Traveling to Europe she was impressed by Toynbee Hall in the slumb of London. In September 1889 she and her college friend, Ellen Gates Star, founded Hull House in Chicago to provide a social center for the poor working people in the neighborhood. This was the beginning of the social settlement movement in the United States. Hull House became a focal point for social reforms in child labor laws, protection of immigrants, labor unions, and working conditions as well as a meeting place for educational and cultural activities. Her excellent book *Twenty Years at Hull House* describes this experience.

In *Newer Ideals of Peace,* published in 1907, Jane Addams criticized the militarism in city government, the inadequate responses of legislation to the needs of an industrial society, the lack of immigrants and women in local government, the inadequate protection of children, and the social problems in the labor movement. Based on her experience in working with immigrants from various countries, she developed a cosmopolitan attitude which she called "cosmic patriotism." She became an ardent internationalist and hoped that people could move beyond their narrow nationalist orientations toward a more universal human effort and affection.

Jane Addams was vice-president of the National American Woman Suffrage Association from 1911 to 1914; but when the war broke out in Europe, she devoted all her energies to working for peace. In September 1914 Rosika Schwimmer, a Hungarian journalist and suffragist, came to America and spoke to President Wilson, Secretary of State Bryan, and then the general public about the United States intervening to negotiate a peace settlement. Emmeline Pethick-Lawrence, an English feminist, spoke at a suffrage rally in Carnegie Hall about organizing a woman's peace movement. Crystal Eastman formed a woman's peace committee and suggested that Pethick-Lawrence contact Jane Addams in Chicago. Carrie Chapman Catt also wrote Jane Addams a letter complaining that "the present management of the peace movement in this country is overmasculinized." Addams agreed that women were the most eager for action, and she and Catt called a national conference of women's organizations.

They gathered in Washington on January 9, 1915 and formed the Woman's Peace Party with a very insightful program. To stop the current war they suggested a conference of delegates from neutral nations or at least an unofficial conference of pacifists. To make sure that the settlement terms would not sow the seeds of new wars they recommended self-determination and autonomy for all disputed territories, no war indemnities unless international law had been violated, and democratic control of foreign policy and treaty arrangements. To secure world peace for the future they suggested the following: a "Concert of Nations" to replace the "balance of power" with an international congress, an international police force, and courts to settle all disputes between nations; an immediate and permanent League of Neutral Nations with binding arbitration, judicial, and legislative procedures and an international police force for protection; progressive national disarmament protected by the peace program; until disarmament is complete the nationalization of munitions manufacture; protection of private property at sea; international and national action to remove the economic causes of war; and the extension of democratic principles of self-government, including woman suffrage. The national program for the United States included approval of the Peace Commission Treaties that require a year's investigation before any declaration of war, protest against the increase of armaments, and a recommendation that the President and U.S. Government set up a commission of men and women to work for the prevention of war.

Three thousand people attended the mass meeting, and Jane Addams was elected chairman. National headquarters was established in Chicago, and within a year 25,000 women had joined. Crystal Eastman felt that the reason for having a Woman's Peace Party "is that women are mothers, or potential mothers, therefore have a more intimate sense of the value of human life and that, therefore, there can be more meaning and passion in the determination of a woman's organization to end war than in an organization of men and women with the same aim."

In an article for *Survey* Crystal Eastman explained how the Woman's Peace Congress at The Hague was organized by the Dutch suffragist Aletta Jacobs, "one of a group of 'international' women who are challenging public opinion with the idea of world union for peace." The Woman Suffrage Alliance meeting scheduled for Berlin had to be cancelled because of the war. Instead, Dr. Jacobs called a meeting in February 1915 at Amsterdam to plan a larger congress of individuals to focus on methods of bringing about peace. Leaders from Belgium, Germany, and Britain met with their Dutch hostesses and issued a call for an international Congress of Women at The Hague on April 28; they invited Jane Addams to preside.

Representatives of over 150 organizations from twelve countries gathered that spring of 1915. 1136 women voted to adopt twenty resolutions. These were similar to the program of the Woman's Peace Party. In addition they decided to urge the neutral countries to offer continuous mediation for a peace settlement between the belligerent nations, and they selected envoys to approach the different governments. Jane Addams, Aletta Jacobs, and the Italian Rosa Genoni went to Austro-Hungary, Belgium, Britain, France, Germany, Italy, and Switzerland. Emily Balch, Chrystal Macmillan, Cor Ramondt-Hirschmann, and Rosika Schwimmer were sent to the Scandinavian countries and Russia. In Sweden alone 343 meetings were held on June 27, and The Hague resolutions were signed by 88,784 women. In August Jane Addams met with President Wilson who said that the resolutions were the best formulation he had seen so far.

Leaders of the belligerent governments declared that they had no objection to a conference of neutral nations, even though they could not ask for mediation. Three out of five neutral European nations were ready to join in such a conference, while the other two were still deliberating. By fall, all the leading belligerent nations were willing to cooperate in a Neutral Conference, and the neutrals Norway, Sweden, Denmark, and Holland were eager to participate if the conference were to be called by the United States. Unfortunately the U.S. declined for the reasons that Latin American countries could not be ignored nor was there room for many of them to participate and that the Central Powers had the technical military advantage at that time. Another neutral country would offer to call the conference if the United States would attend, but this made no difference. Even 10,000 telegrams to President Wilson from woman's organizations were of no avail.

In January 1916 the Woman's Peace Party became the United States section of the international organization which came to be named the Women's International League for Peace and Freedom. Henry Ford donated a chartered ship to take women to Europe for a private Neutral Conference which was held in Stockholm on January 26. They formulated further appeals to the neutral and belligerent nations to begin mediation.

Crystal Eastman started in November 1915 the "Truth About Preparedness Campaign" sponsored by the Woman's Peace Party and the American Union Against Militarism. She revealed the economic exploitation behind the industrialists' propaganda for military increases through public debates and numerous articles. In the summer of 1916 AUAM's private investigation of the facts in Mexico and massive publicity campaign prevented the United States from entering into a misguided war with Mexico. In 1917 Crystal Eastman and Roger Baldwin founded the American Civil Liberties Union to protect human rights. After America entered the war, Eastman and other radicals struggled for an early peace, opposed conscription, universal military training, and other repressive legislation; they sponsored classes led by pacifists such as Norman Angell and Emily Green Balch.

Disappointed by Wilson's entering into the war, Jane Addams turned her efforts to the struggle for food. She urged international cooperation and demanded that food blockades, still in place after the armistice, be immediately lifted. She felt that women could do much for international organization especially in regard to such a basic issue as food for survival.

In 1919 the International Congress of Women held in Zurich criticized the peace terms for sanctioning secret agreements, denying self-determination, giving spoils to the victors, creating discord in Europe, demanding disarmament only for the losing side, and condemning a hundred million people to poverty, disease, despair, hatred, and anarchy because of the economic proposals. They welcomed a League of Nations, which four years earlier had seemed so unrealistic to many, but they criticized the plan for varying from Wilson's fourteen points.

As the League of Nations was forming, the Women's International League for Peace and Freedom (WILPF) established its headquarters in Geneva where they kept a close watch on the League of Nations Assembly and Secretariat. WILPF helped to publicize its proceedings and offered frequent criticism. In lectures Jane Addams urged the United States to participate in the World Court. In 1924 WILPF suggested that governments agree to the compulsory jurisdiction of the Permanent Court of International Justice. Their Congress held in Washington that year also recommended better education to avoid mass-suggestion, the abolition of capital punishment and the improvement of prisons, and a better balance of influence between men and women.

The 1929 WILPF Congress in Prague warned that modern warfare threatened civilian populations and that the only way to safety is disarmament. The Zurich Congress of 1934 formulated aims that became WILPF policy for the next quarter century. The primary goals read: "Total and universal disarmament, the abolition of violent means of coercion for the settlement of all conflicts, the substitution in every case of some form of peaceful settlement, and the development of a world organization for the political, social and economic co-operation of peoples." In addition they committed themselves to studying and alleviating the causes of war by nonviolent social reform.

When Chamberlain appeased Hitler in 1938 at Munich, WILPF issued this strong response:

It is a sham peace based on the violation of law, justice and right. It is a so-called 'peaceful change' dictated by four Powers and forced upon a young and small State, which was not represented when its dismemberment was finally decided upon.

The International Chairmen of WILPF sent out an appeal to help Czechoslovakia financially and economically. In it they declared that pacifism is "not the quietistic acceptance of betrayal and lies" but the struggle for truth, right, clear political aims, and the "courageous initiative for a constructive policy of just peace."

In 1951 WILPF considered a plan for a nonviolent national defense along Gandhian lines to deter aggression without the disadvantages and dangers of armaments. They discovered that the following nonviolent principles must be understood by the people before this can work on a national scale:

Recognition that violence breeds violence; upholding truth before prestige; acceptance of the principle of equal rights; freedom of conscience and of information; strengthening of altruistic rather than materialistic values.

In recent years WILPF has supported the United Nations, and criticized the Korean War, nuclear arms and testing, civil rights violations, the Vietnam War, and the nuclear arms race. In March 1983 WILPF representatives visited the NATO governments to protest the deployment of more nuclear weapons in Europe. WILPF remains perhaps the largest, most international and influential of all the women's peace organizations.

Another great peacemaker and social reformer was Dorothy Day of the Catholic Worker. Dorothy was born in Brooklyn on November 8, 1897. A scholarship helped her to attend the University of Illinois where she joined a socialist group. Her family moved back to New York, and she was soon mixing as a writer and activist with Eugene O'Neill, John Reed, Louise

Bryant, and Max Eastman. She wrote for *The Masses* until it was suppressed.

In 1917 she went to Washington to picket the White House with the suffragists. She was arrested and bailed out. When the thirty-five of them appeared in court, they were convicted; but their sentencing was postponed. That afternoon they picketed and were arrested again, going through the same procedure. The third time they refused to pay bail. The leaders were sentenced to six months, the older women to fifteen days, and the rest, including Dorothy, to thirty days. They demanded to be treated as political prisoners and went on a hunger strike for ten days until their demands were met.

For many years Dorothy Day worked as a free-lance writer. She published a novel and even sold its movie rights. She raised her daughter, and in 1928 she became a Catholic. She and Peter Maurin began the Catholic Worker movement in the depths of the depression. They began publishing a newspaper called *The Catholic Worker* in May 1933. About twenty people moved into a house on the west side of New York; they fed the hungry and clothed the needy. Soon "houses of hospitality" were being started in Boston, Rochester, Milwaukee, and other cities. They lived in voluntary poverty, practicing Christ's teachings.

During World War II Day wrote in *The Catholic Worker* about the immorality of conscription, and she urged Catholics to be conscientious objectors. In 1955 she organized a civil disobedience protest against New York City's compulsory air raid drill. Each year a small group spent a few days in jail for this purpose. "We wanted to act against war and getting ready for war: nerve gas, germ warfare, guided missiles, testing and stockpiling of nuclear bombs, conscription, the collection of income tax — against the entire militarism of the state." They did this every year until in 1961, after 2,000 people refused to take shelter, the city decided to drop the requirement.

On April 22, 1963 the Mothers for Peace, a group made up of Catholic Workers, members of Pax, Women Strike for Peace, WILPF, the Fellowship of Reconciliation, and others, met with Pope John XXIII to plead for a condemnation of nuclear war and the development of nonviolent resistance. Dorothy Day also participated in the civil rights movement at this time, traveling to Danville, Virginia to pray, march, boycott, and suffer imprisonment for the rights of black people. During the Vietnam War she inspired the radical Catholic Left to protest. She continued to oppose conscription and taxes for war, and in 1965 she spoke at a draft card burning. At the age of 75 she was arrested for picketing with Cesar Chavez and the United Farm Workers Union and spent twelve days in jail. The continuing Catholic Worker movement is her great legacy.

The tremendous influence of feminism on the peace movement in the sixties and seventies is perhaps best typified by Barbara Deming. Writing for *The Nation* and *Liberation* magazines she described her participation in various nonviolent protest movements. She visited Cuba and North Vietnam and reported the viewpoints of the other side. She explained the philosophy and methods of the Committee for Nonviolent Action (CNVA) and their recommendation of unilateral disarmament to all countries including the Soviet Union. In her account of the San Francisco to Moscow walk the mirror images of Russian and American fears and defense policies were revealed. At the same time the person-to-person effectiveness of nonviolent direct action was eloquently portrayed. By walking for peace in the South she combined the quest for civil rights and justice with peace and nonviolence. She was arrested for civil disobedience in Birmingham, Alabama and Albany, Georgia. During the Vietnam War she lectured and wrote about the atrocities the United States was perpetrating against the Vietnamese people. She particularly pointed out the Lazy Dog bombs that are ineffective against the "steel and concrete" targets but are designed to enter flesh. She told of how schools, hospitals, and homes were being bombed unmercifully.

Barbara Deming became a strong advocate of nonviolent revolution as the most effective way to transform a violent and oppressive society. Although she sympathizes with revolutionaries who feel the need for violent methods of liberation, she argues that in nonviolent struggle there will be fewer casualties. She acknowledges that in standing up to violent power, some suffering is inevitable. Yet she believes that the nonviolent action of assertive noncooperation with the oppressors can be as strong and effective as violent struggle while maintaining the respect for everyone's human rights. She writes, "This is how we stand up for ourselves nonviolently: we refuse the authorities our labor, we refuse them our money (our taxes), we refuse them our bodies (to fight in their wars). We strike." She goes on to recommend blocking, obstructing, and disrupting the operation of a system in which people are not free. At the same time the adversary is confronted, his rights are respected, and he is made to examine his conscience about what is just. A violent response to a nonviolent action further reveals the injustice and loses sympathy from allies and supporters. Deming believes that nonviolent methods have barely begun to be used with their full power.

Like Andrea Dworkin, Deming came to believe that nonviolence must be combined with radical feminism, for the patriarchal male dominance over submissive women pervades the entire society in deeply ingrained ways. Women and everyone in the peace movement must insist on the equality of the sexes and live the revolution in their personal lives. Feminism and pacifism have much in common. Caroline Wildflower describes how feminism has improved the peace movement. She describes how in the sixties the male leaders were reluctant to give women shared leadership. Instead, women were assigned to secretarial work. When the Women's Movement started raising the consciousness about these injustices in society, changes began to happen in spite of the resistance of habit. Not only were the authorities and hierarchies of society being challenged, but the same structures within the peace groups were being scrutinized and criticized by empowered women. The results of this continuing evolution are that the group processes are becoming more egalitarian, jobs are rotated so that everyone is broadened, women are expressing an equal voice with more emotional power, men are becoming more sensitive to their own feminine qualities, and a more healthy overall balance is emerging.

In the eighties the military buildup under President Reagan is stimulating the peace movement to mobilize. Women, minorities, and the poor have been neglected while the Pentagon budget accelerates. The issues have become especially obvious to women when increased expenditures on nuclear weapons, missiles, bombers, submarines, aircraft carriers, etc. are compared to decreases in education, health, job training, family aid, food, housing, energy, civil rights, environmental protection, etc. The five-year military budget for the U.S. alone is projected at 1.6 trillion dollars. World military expenditures average $19,300 per soldier while public education spending averages $380 per student. The governmental budgets of the Western powers allot four times as much money to military research as they do to health research. The world in 1982 spent 1800 times as much on military forces as it did on international peacekeeping. In April 1982 the Women's Pentagon Action Unity Statement included the following:

> Our cities are in ruin, bankrupt; they suffer the devastation of war. Hospitals are closed, our schools deprived of books and teachers. Our Black and Latino youth are without decent work. They will be forced, drafted to become cannon fodder for the very power that oppresses them. Whatever help the poor receive is cut or withdrawn to feed the Pentagon which needs about $500,000,000 a day for its murderous health . . . We women are gathering because life on the precipice is intolerable.

Many women, such as Ann Davidon, speak about breaking through the "macho mental barrier" and demilitarizing society by shifting resources to useful production. Sally Gearhart believes "the rising up of women in this century to be the human race's response to the threat of its own self-annihilation and the destruction of the planet." She calls upon the world's women to take the responsibility for sustaining life.

The women's peace movement is truly international. In October 1981 over a thousand women from 133 countries met in Prague, Czechoslovakia on the themes Equality, National Independence, and Peace. They all agreed that the nuclear arms race must be stopped and that women and men of good will can prevent nuclear war. The Women's International Democratic

Federation (WIDF) reports on the activities of the women's peace movement in Europe and the Soviet Union. Hundreds of thousands of women are protesting the danger of war, not only in western Europe but in eastern Europe and the Soviet Union as well. The Soviet Women's Committee reports that during the last week of October 1982 Action for Disarmament was celebrated in the USSR by fifty million people with over 80,000 events in protest of the arms race. According to WIDF, in the spring of 1982 women demonstrated for peace in Angola, Argentina, Australia, Belgium, Canada, Czechoslovakia, Finland, West Germany (800,000 citizens), East Germany (77,000 women), Great Britain (100,000), Greece, Italy, Japan (30,000 in Tokyo on Easter), Jemen, Mauritius, Mozambique (20,000 women), Nicaragua (100,000), Netherlands, New Zealand (20,000 women), Poland, Soviet Union, Sweden, and the USA. Women's peace camps have been established at Greenham Common in England and at Seneca, New York.

If men through their aggression, power urges, and rigid stubbornness have caused war after war, then women through their love, nurturing, and flexibility can help us to learn how to prevent wars in order to save our civilization. Western civilization in the twentieth century has become pathologically destructive, endangering all life. Much therapy and healing is needed to cure the disease of masculine militarism. Feminist nonviolence is clearly the remedy recommended by the greatest of the peacemakers. Our society as a whole and each person individually must learn to revere the loving, sensitive, caring, empathetic qualities of our being. Women are excellent teachers of peace in this process that will evolve into a balanced, healthy, integrated, and just society. Feminism has enabled women to take their rightful place in the anti-nuclear movement, thus strengthening the power and health of the peace movement.

The Anti-Nuclear Movement

"In the name of God, let us abolish nuclear weapons."
The New Abolitionist Covenant

"We are the curators of life on earth,
standing at a crossroads in time.
We must awake from our false sense of security
and commit ourselves to using democracy constructively
to save the human species."

Helen Caldicott

"We reject violence completely,
because the structural violence caused by this decision
to place these missiles or to continue the arms race
on both sides is violence."

Petra Kelly

"To end the danger of nuclear war the nations must
not merely freeze nuclear weapons but abolish them."

Randal Forsberg

"We must protest if we are to survive.
Protest is the only realistic form of civil defense."

E.P. Thompson

The empowerment of women is exemplified in the anti-nuclear movement by three of its most important voices: Helen Caldicott, Randall Forsberg, and Petra Kelly. Although protests against the use of nuclear technology began with its inception when Leo Szilard and seventy scientists petitioned President Truman not to use the atomic bomb on the Japanese, the focus of this chapter is on the anti-nuclear movement which has grown tremendously in the late seventies and early eighties.

Demonstrations against nuclear power plants in western Europe began in France and West Germany in 1971. Protests increased, and in February 1975 a major breakthrough for the anti-nuclear movement occurred in Wyhl of southwestern Germany. When construction of the power plant was about to begin, several hundred local activists (farmers, housewives, merchants, students) held a press conference at the construction site and sat down in front of the bulldozers. Police cleared the area by using water cannons and arresting people. Nevertheless, some local people stayed there overnight, and they returned the next week with 28,000 supporters from all over Germany and from Alsace in France. People occupied the land for over a year and operated a school to educate people on nuclear issues. They agreed to leave when a panel of judges was established, and in 1977 the panel ruled against the plant.

During the summer of 1976 the construction site for a nuclear power plant at Seabrook, New Hampshire was occupied by 180 people, and the following April more than 2,000 members of the Clamshell Alliance marched onto the site where construction had begun. On the first of May 1,414 people were arrested at the Seabrook site. The Clams were well organized into affinity groups of 10-20 people who were trained in nonviolence and practiced consensus decision making. They attempted to avoid a hierarchical and authoritarian leadership structure by letting every person in each group and each group within the whole participate in the process. Of those arrested, more than half refused to pay bail and stayed in custody for two weeks.

The example of the Clamshell Alliance stimulated a more active resistance in California to the almost completed Diablo Canyon nuclear reactors. In June 1977 the Abalone Alliance was formed. The Mothers For Peace had filed as intervenors in 1973 and were glad to see the effort mobilizing. Nonviolence was strictly adhered to when 47 people were arrested for trespassing on August 7, 1977. One year later 487 occupiers and blockaders were arrested for their civil disobedience. The Abalone Alliance adopted the feminist process of consensus and the affinity group structure.

By the time fuel-loading was due to begin in September 1981 an excellent handbook had been published to educate new activists on the processes; numerous affinity groups were prepared from all over California; and the direct action was extended for two weeks with nearly two thousand arrests. Shortly after the action, numerous errors were discovered in the plans and buildings of the plant, and two years later the plant was still not close to becoming operational.

For many people, including myself, the experience at Diablo Canyon in the encampment, the nonviolence training, the affinity group friendship, the consensus processes, the arrest, and the time together in jail were deeply moving and inspiring. The Nonviolence Code, which was agreed to by every affinity group, was as follows: "1) Our attitude will be one of openness, friendliness, and respect towards all people we encounter. 2) We will use no violence, verbal or physical, toward any person. 3) We will not damage any property. 4) We will not bring or use any drugs or alcohol other than for medical purposes. 5) We will not run. 6) We will carry no weapons." These Nonviolence Guidelines have been adopted by various direct actions in California sponsored by the Livermore Action Group, the Vandenberg Action Coalition, and others.

At Diablo Canyon in 1981 strong solidarity was achieved on refusing to pay any money for bail or fines and also on refusing to accept probation. Most people were released after four days for time served, but over five hundred people became defendants represented by Richard Frischman using the defense of necessity argument — that people had to act out of a moral necessity in order to prevent a greater harm or danger. This case is still pending, and the defense of necessity is being used by increasing numbers of anti-nuclear activists in order to challenge these evils through the judicial process.

During my week in jail I got to know the white-haired Bob Schneider from Berkeley; he now goes by the name of Eldred. He told me that this Diablo action was so fantastic that he wanted to help organize the same thing at the Livermore Laboratory in northern California where research for nuclear weapons is conducted. I agreed that the danger of nuclear weapons is even greater than that of nuclear power. In February 1982 the Livermore Action Group had their first action, and on June 21 of that year 1,400 blockaders disrupted business as usual at the lab and were arrested. That same month 1,691 blockaded the United Nations offices of the nuclear weapons powers, and nearly a million people marched in the streets of New York for nuclear disarmament.

In 1978 hundreds of people had been arrested over a period of eight months at Rocky Flats, Colorado where nuclear bombs are made. Daniel Ellsberg called Rocky Flats the Auschwitz of our time. The movie "In the King of Prussia" portrays the trial of Dan and Philip Berrigan and six others of the "Plowshares 8" for hammering on the Mark 12A nosecones (a first-strike weapon) at a General Electric plant in Pennsylvania.

The conversion of two Catholic bishops, Matthiesen in Amarillo, Texas and Hunthausen of Seattle, was stimulated by personal contact with individuals arrested for civil disobedience. Matthiesen is urging workers to quit Pantex where nuclear weapons are assembled, and Hunthausen is withholding income taxes from the Federal government to protest military spending. Jim and Shelley Douglass, who influenced Bishop Hunthausen in Washington, have organized a group called Ground Zero, which has protested Trident submarines since 1975 and in 1983 the white train carrying nuclear weapons. Their dual focus in their nonviolent civil disobedience campaign is Christ's kingdom of God and international law.

The Los Angeles Catholic Workers, who operate a free soup kitchen on skid row to feed about 800 people a day, have been active in civil disobedience for several years protesting nuclear weapons businesses in southern California. Following in Dorothy Day's tradition, Jeff Dietrich, Catherine Morris, and others have been arrested several times.

The planned flight testing of the MX missile at Vandenberg Air Force Base on the central coast of California brought protestors from all over the state in January and March of 1983. About 200 were arrested and banned from the base in the first action. Many of these people returned in March and were joined by hundreds more who stayed in jail a week in solidarity for equal sentences; in this second action 800 were arrested. Congress had delayed some of the MX missile funds, which were to be voted on again in May. That month Jim Wallis of the Sojourners led 242 Christians into the halls of the U.S. Congress to pray; they were arrested for an illegal demonstration. On June 17 the first MX missile flight test occurred at Vandenberg while protestors were being arrested on the base. The Vandenberg Action Coalition is just one of the many activist groups that have sprung up around the world.

Since the missile flights are targeted at the Marshall Islands, these protestants are connected to the efforts of Pacific Islanders for a nuclear-free Pacific.

The Livermore Action Group (LAG) of Berkeley initiated the first annual International Day of Nuclear Disarmament on June 20, 1983. On that day legal rallies and nonviolent civil disobedience occurred in over fifty locations across the United States. At Livermore alone over a thousand people were arrested. Most of them refused to be arraigned because they would not accept probation; after a week the judge relented on the probation. The objectives of this action were as follows: "To further the causes of: 1) global nuclear disarmament, 2) demilitarization and nonintervention, 3) equitable distribution of wealth and resources within and among nations, and 4) a sustainable relationship between the human race and the planet. To protest, halt, and disrupt the design, production, transport, and deployment of nuclear weapons worldwide for at least one working day."

In West Germany the anti-nuclear and ecology movements have grown into a full-fledged political party — the Greens. They have managed to combine direct action protests with electoral politics, and in March 1983 the Green Party captured 27 seats in the national Parliament. As their most articulate spokesperson in English, Petra Kelly, has pointed out, one of their main concerns is the U.S. deployment of Pershing II and cruise missiles in western Europe scheduled to begin in December 1983.

The anti-nuclear movement is active throughout western Europe, while in eastern Europe it primarily has to operate through official organizations. In England more than a dozen peace camps have been established, Greenham Common being the most well-known. European Nuclear Disarmament (END) under the leadership of E.P. Thompson has grown tremendously in a few years.

One of the most unusual aspects of the anti-nuclear movement, particularly in California, is the egalitarian methods of shifting roles and leadership positions so that many people can develop leadership skills. In fact most people shy away from the word "leader," preferring the role names of facilitator or spokesperson.

Feminist awareness and consensus process attempt to be sensitive to every person's feelings, and the effort is always to keep a sense of group unity by resolving dissension. Yet every person and each group is considered autonomous. One group or even one person in a group can block consensus if there is an ethical objection to an action. Actually it is a moral responsibility to protest an immoral action which may affect the group. This is in reality the basis of civil disobedience toward a society which is allowing immoral actions. As with Gandhi, people in the anti-nuclear movement feel that the means is as important as the end. Therefore a great emphasis is placed on the purity of the process. When affinity groups of five to fifteen people all agree on something, and when a spokes-council of representatives from those groups all achieve a unanimous decision involving hundreds of people, the moral and spiritual power of the resulting action can be awesome. Through this process of alternating spokes-council and affinity group meetings, goals are determined, strategies and tactics develop and change, and virtually every decision important to the group is made in such a way that every individuial can influence the result.

At the same time as the nonvioilent direct action movement has been growing, a nation-wide campaign in the United States for serious nuclear arms control has developed a ground-swell of support through the bilateral nuclear weapons freeze proposal. The Freeze was conceived in the summer of 1979 when the American Friends Service Committee proposed a "Nuclear Moratorium" and arms control scholar Randall Forsberg wrote an essay on "Confining the Military to Defense as a Route to Disarmament" in which she suggested that both the USA and USSR stop producing nuclear weapons as a first step. This idea struck a chord with leaders in the peace movement when she spoke at the Mobilization for Survival annual convention in September. Encouraged by them she wrote up her proposal in a four-page "Call to Halt the Arms Race." The following paragraph from that document was to become the basis of Freeze resolutions all around the country:

To improve national and international security, the United States and the Soviet Union should stop the nuclear arms race. Specifically, they should adopt a mutual freeze on the testing, production and deployment of nuclear weapons and of missiles and new aircraft designed primarily to deliver nuclear weapons. This is an essential, verifiable first step toward lessening the risk of nuclear war and reducing the nuclear arsenals.

Senator Mark Hatfield introduced in the U.S. Senate an amendment to the SALT II treaty calling for a Freeze, and in January 1980 a conference of about 30 peace groups endorsed Forsberg's Freeze proposal. The Freeze resolution was placed on the ballot in 62 cities and towns in Massachusetts, and in November it passed in all but three; the Freeze even passed in 30 where Reagan also won. In 1981 Freeze resolutions were endorsed by the legislatures of Massachusetts, Oregon, New York, Connecticut, Maine, Minnesota, Vermont, Wisconsin, Kansas, Iowa, and Maryland.

Senators Kennedy and Hatfield introduced a Freeze resolution in March 1982 and immediately attracted 25 co-sponsors in the Senate and 125 in the House of Representatives. Although 60-85% of the American people favored a Freeze, pressure against it from two thousand corporate lobbyists led to its narrow defeat in the House on August 5 by a vote of 204 to 202. However, in the 1982 elections Nuclear Freeze Initiatives were passed by the people in California, Massachusetts, Michigan, Montana, New Jersey, North Dakota, Oregon, Rhode Island, Chicago, Denver, Philadelphia, Washington D.C., and Dade County. For the first time in history as many as 18 million people voted on the issue of nuclear weapons; 60% of them voted for the Freeze, even though President Reagan opposed it. In seventy Congressional races where the Freeze was a key issue, pro-Freeze candidates won in 64% of them. On May 4, 1983 the U.S. House of Representatives passed the Freeze resolution 278-149.

A bilateral nuclear weapons freeze that is verifiable is an excellent proposal at this time, because the Soviet Union has just recently caught up to parity with the United States in military power. Yet the Reagan Administration is attempting to forge ahead to military superiority again by developing and deploying new first-strike weapons such as the Trident II, MX, Pershing II, and cruise missiles. A complete Freeze would also be a comprehensive test ban and would be easier to verify than SALT I or II, according to Herbert Scoville, former Deputy Director of the Central Intelligence Agency. Common sense tells us that the arms race must be stopped before it can be reversed.

The Freeze campaign has become a national, mainstream issue, and much of the effort behind it has come from professional organizations such as the Physicians for Social Responsibility which was led for four years by Dr. Helen Caldicott. In her care for children's health as a pediatrician and as a native of Australia in the south Pacific, Caldicott has been concerned for a long time about the medical dangers of radioactivity. Her lectures, films, and books on nuclear madness have stirred thousands of anti-nuclear activists. In 1979 she organized a symposium of experts on the subject of "The Medical Consequences of Nuclear War" which addressed large audiences in major cities across the United States. A short film showing the highlights of the symposium called "The Last Epidemic" has been shown by peace groups and Freeze advocates to thousands of small groups. Another film of one of Caldicott's moving lectures on the nuclear arms issue, "If You Love this Planet," won the Academy Award.

Caldicott is not afraid to use strong and deep emotions of concern for the survival of our human civilization in order to stir her listeners to action. She considers this issue of human survival to be the ultimate issue of all time. Her latest endeavor is to start a women's survival party; the symbol for it is a baby.

Her work stimulated the forming of the International Physicians for the Prevention of Nuclear War, and in the fall of 1982 they presented a television program that was shown uncensored in both the Soviet Union and the United States. Three Soviet physicians and three American physicians all agreed that the only cure for nuclear war was prevention and the elimination of nuclear weapons.

An indication of how widespread and diverse the peace movement has become can be seen by the various professional organizations that have been spiringing up so rapidly. They include the Educators for Social Responsibility, Lawyers Committee for Nuclear Policy, High Technology Professionals for Peace, Lawyers Alliance for Nuclear Arms Control, Union of Concerned Scientists, Business Executives for National Security, Architects for Social Responsibility, Social Workers for Peace and Nuclear Disarmament, Union of Concerned Psychoanalysts and Psychotherapists, Artists for Survival, and many others.

Religious and church groups have become more active than ever. The Catholic bishops, the World Council of Churches, and many other church denominations, including the Lutherans in East Germany, are offering strong criticisms of the nuclear arms race.

In fact it is practically impossible to keep up with all of the contemporary organizing to struggle for a secure peace in the world. I hope the reader will forgive me for the sketchiness of this information. By the time this book is published, so much more will already be happening. Although the major media of television, radio, newspapers, and magazines cover very little of the peace movement activities around the world, the people who are working for peace are discovering each other through alternate media. Thousands of people are being touched in personal ways every day, and a momentum is building which can and must lead to global change from an arms race and militarization to disarmament and nonviolent methods of resolving conflicts.

Conclusions: What Can We Do?

From the ancient sages and mystics to modern political activists, the essential reality of a life of peace has not changed. Love for our fellow beings is always superior to hatred and fear. Nonviolence has been the method of the greatest peacemakers. Philosophers of vision have seen the need for the unity of human beings so that differences can be settled by intelligent means. Human civilization is evolving steadily toward a federal world government which can provide institutions to settle conflicts between nations in humane ways. The sophistication of scientific technology applied as military force has created an inescapable crisis for the human species which must be solved one way or another. Total war has become inseparable from mass suicide. To survive, human beings must learn self-restraint and less destructive means of resolving conflict. In the 1980s the complete devastation of the northern hemisphere depends on the hair-triggers in the hands of the United States' and the Soviet Union's political leaders. Those leaders and the military industrial complexes which support their power have a vested interest in maintaining and increasing their military power. Yet they are the leaders of their nations, because the people allow them to lead by supporting them. Therefore it is up to the people to recognize the danger to their lives and the future of the earth and to demand life-affirming policies from their governments.

This is where every person has the opportunity and the responsibility to influence the course of our civilization for the good of all. It does not take a great philosopher to understand that peace and justice in the world would be for the good of all, while war and oppression benefit a few at the expense of many. Some individuals are becoming more aware of the true means to peace through nonviolence and a system of justice for everyone in the world. Yet many people are still hypnotized by political leaders who use national pride and the fear of foreign powers to manipulate people for selfish interests.

Now that we are poised on the brink of a nuclear holocaust, the time has come for the good people and the goodness in all people to rise up and demonstrate a peaceful way to achieve a stable

259

peace. The threat of nuclear deterrence is too dangerous to offer a permanent peace, but it is allowing a breathing spell from all-out war so that better methods can be developed. War can break out suddenly, but peacemaking takes time, patience, education, and communication. Before the political leaders will give up their use of nationalistic military methods to try to solve problems, enough people must be educated to understand better methods. As those people demonstrate the effectiveness of nonviolent methods, a democratic process of change will occur. Then the peace-loving people can lead the world toward a stable system of international law that respects the rights of everyone.

You who are reading this book are probably more enlightened on these points than most. Those who truly realize that love and understanding are more effective in peacemaking than hatred and force are the people who will be changing the world for the better by communicating and educating others. As Einstein clearly saw, what is needed is a chain reaction of awareness from person to person to person. Once the truth is known in one's heart, there is no way it can be unlearned. In this time of awful danger for our planet, everyone has a moral obligation to act in some way to save humanity from the horrible designs of the hateful, the fearful, the selfish, and the greedy.

Each person has the ability to hear the voice of conscience in one's own heart. Each person knows best how he or she can contribute to building a peaceful world. The inner guidance is always with us, beckoning us on toward greater challenges. The great peacemakers have demonstrated various ways of peace, and the philosophers of peace have taught us how peace can be attained. Everyone can help. This is our life, and the future is in our hands. The ultimate conclusions are the actions we take individually and collectively. Let us work together to create a world of peace and justice.

Bibliography

1. Chinese Sages: Lao Tzu, Confucius, Mo Tzu, and Mencius
Chan, Wing-tsit *A Source Book in Chinese Philosophy*.
Confucius *Confucian Analects, The Great Learning & The Doctrine of the Mean* tr. James Legge.
Confucius, The Analects of tr. Arthur Waley.
The Sacred Books of Confucius and Other Confucian Classics ed. and tr. Ch'u Chai and Winberg Chai.
Lao Tsu *Tao Te Ching* tr. Gia-fu Feng and Jane English.
Lin Yutang (ed.) *The Wisdom of India and China*.
Motse, The Ethical and Political Works of tr. Yi-pao Mei.
Mo. Tzu *Basic Writings* tr. Burton Watson.
Welch, Holmes *Taoism: The Parting of the Way*.

2. Indian Mystics: Mahavira and the Buddha
Coomaraswamy, Ananda *Buddha and the Gospel of Buddhism*.
Jaina Sutras tr. Hermann Jacobi.
Lin Yutang (ed.) *The Wisdom of China and India*.
Noss, John B. *Man's Religions*.
Radhakrishnan, Sarvepalli and Charles A. Moore *A Source Book in Indian Philosophy*.
The Thirteen Principal Upanishads tr. Robert Ernest Hume.
Zimmer, Heinrich *Philosophies of India*.

3. Greek Conscience: Pythagoras, Socrates, and Aristophanes
Aristophanes *Plays* tr. Benjamin Bickley Rogers.
Diogenes Laertius *Lives of Eminent Philosophers* tr. R. D. Hicks.
Kirk, G. S. and J. E. Raven *The Presocratic Philosophers*.
Plato *Dialogues* tr. B. Jowett.
Pythagoras *Golden Verses and Other Fragments*.
Schuré, Edouard *The Great Initiates* tr. Gloria Rasberry.
Watters, Hallie *The Pythagorean Way of Life*.
Xenophon *Memorabilia* tr. E. C. Marchant.
Zampaglione, Gerardo *The Idea of Peace in Antiquity* tr. Richard Dunn.

4. Jesus and the Early Christians
Instead of Violence ed. Arthur and Lila Weinberg.
Levi *The Aquarian Gospel of Jesus the Christ.*
The New Testament.
Zampaglione, Gerardo *The Idea of Peace in Antiquity* tr.
  Richard Dunn.

5. St. Francis of Assisi and The Magna Charta
Costain, Thomas *The Conquering Family (A History of the*
  Plantagenets Vol. I).
Jorgensen, Johannes *Saint Francis of Assisi* tr. T. O'Coner
  Sloane.
The Little Flowers of Saint Francis of Assisi tr. Abby
  Langdon Alger.
Sticco, Maria *The Peace of St. Francis* tr. Salvator Attanasio.

6. Dante on One Government and Chaucer on Counseling
  Peace
Chaucer, Geoffrey *The Canterbury Tales* tr. J. U. Nicolson.
Dante Alighieri *Monarchy and Three Political Letters*
  tr. Donald Nicholl.
Dubois, Pierre *The Recovery of the Holy Land* tr. Walther
  J. Brandt.
Durant, Will *The Age of Faith.*
Gardner, John *The Life and Times of Chaucer.*
Hoover, Herbert and Hugh Gibson *The Problems of Lasting*
  Peace.
Machiavelli, Niccolo *History of Florence.*

7. Erasmus and Humanism
Adams, Robert P. *The Better Part of Valor:* More, Erasmus,
  Colet, and Vives, on Humanism, War, and Peace,
  1496-1535.
Durant, Will *The Reformation.*
The Essential Erasmus tr. John P. Dolan.
Mayer, Peter (ed.) *The Pacifist Conscience.*
Woodward, William Harrison *Studies in Education during*
  the Age of the Renaissance 1400-1600.

Zweig, Stefan *Erasmus of Rotterdam* tr. Eden and Cedar
Paul.

8. Crucé's Peace Plan and Grotius on International Law
Crucé, Eméric *The New Cineas* tr. C. Frederick Farrell, Jr.
and Edith R. Farrell.
Grotius *The Rights of War and Peace* including the Law
of Nature and of Nations, tr. A. C. Campbell; Intro.
by David J. Hill.
Grotius, Hugo *The Rights of War and Peace* tr. and Intro.
by W. S. M. Knight.
Hinsley, F. H. *Power and the Pursuit of Peace:* Theory
and Practice in the History of Relations between
States.
Sully *Grand Design of Henry IV* Intro. by David Ogg.
White, Andrew Dickson *Seven Great Statesmen* in the
Warfare of Humanity with Unreason.

9. George Fox, William Penn and Friends
Brock, Peter *Pacifism in Europe to 1914.*
Brock, Peter *Pioneers of the Peaceable Kingdom.*
The Journal of George Fox a revised edition by John L.
Nickalls.
Knowles, G. W. *Quakers and Peace.*
Passages from the Life and Writings of William Penn,
collected by the editor from his published works and
correspondence and from the biographies of Clarkson,
Lewis, and Janney, and other reliable sources.
Penn, William *The Peace of Europe: The Fruits of Solitude*
and other writings.
Wildes, Harry Emerson *Voice of the Lord:* A Biography
of George Fox.
Wildes, Harry Emerson *William Penn.*
Yolen, Jane *Friend:* The Story of George Fox and the
Quakers.

10. Federalist Peace Plans of Rousseau, Bentham, and Kant
Bentham, Jeremy *An Introduction to the Principles of
Morals and Legislation.*

The Works of Jeremy Bentham Volume II, ed. John Bowring.

Blanchard, William H. *Rousseau and the Spirit of Revolt: A Psychological Study.*

Crocker, Lester G. *Jean-Jacques Rousseau:* The Quest (1712-1758).

French Utopias: An Anthology of Ideal Societies, ed. Frank E. Manuel and Fritzie P. Manuel.

Hinsley, F. H. *Power and the Pursuit of Peace.*

Josephson, Matthew *Jean-Jacques Rousseau.*

Kant, Immanuel *The Critique of Pure Reason* tr. J. M. D. Meiklejohn.

Kant, Immanuel *On History* tr. and ed. Lewis White Beck.

Kant, Immanuel *Lectures on Ethics* tr. Louis Infield.

Kant, Immanuel *Perpetual Peace* tr. with Intro. by M. Campbell Smith.

Kant, Immanuel *The Science of Right* tr. W. Hastie.

Mack, Mary P. *Jeremy Bentham:* An Odyssey of Ideas 1748-1792.

Perkins, Merle L. *The Moral and Political Philosophy of the Abbe de Saint-Pierre.*

The Confessions of Jean Jacques Rousseau.

Rousseau, Jean Jacques *A Discourse on the Origin of Inequality, A Discourse on Political Economy, The Social Contract* tr. G. D. H. Cole.

Rousseau, Jean-Jacques *Emile or On Education* tr. Allan Bloom.

Rousseau, Jean Jacques *A Lasting Peace through the Federation of Europe* tr. C. E. Vaughan.

11. Emerson's Transcendentalism and Thoreau's Civil Disobedience

Brooks, Van Wyck *The Life of Emerson.*

Canby, Henry Seidel *Thoreau.*

Channing, William Ellery *Discourses on War.*

The Complete Writings of Ralph Waldo Emerson.

Huggard, William Allen *Emerson and the Problem of War and Peace.*

The Journal of Henry D. Thoreau ed. Bradford Torrey and Francis H. Allen.

Thoreau, Henry D. *Reform Papers* ed. Wendell Glick.
Thoreau, Henry D. *The Annotated Walden* ed. Philip Van Doren Stern.
Thoreau, Henry David *The Variorum Walden and the Variorum Civil Disobedience* ed. Walter Harding.

12. Religion for World Peace: Bahá'u'lláh and 'Abdu'l-Bahá
'Abdu'l-Bahá *Foundations of World Unity.*
Bahá'u'lláh and 'Abdu'l-Bahá *Bahá'í World Faith.*
The Proclamation of Bahá'u'lláh to the kings and leaders of the world.
Bahá'u'lláh *The Seven Valleys and the Four Valleys* tr. Marzieh Gail and Ali-Kuli Khan.
Esslemont, J. E. *Bahá'u'lláh and the New Era.*
Shogi, Effendi *The Dispensation of Bahá'u'lláh.*

13. Leo Tolstoy on the Law of Love
Hofmann, Modest and Andre Pierre *By Deeds of Truth: The Life of Leo Tolstoy.*
Tolstoy, Leo *A Confession, The Gospel in Brief, and What I Believe* tr. Aylmer Maude.
Tolstoy, Leo *The Kingdom of God Is Within You* tr. Leo Wiener.
Tolstoy, Leo *The Law of Love and the Law of Violence* tr. Mary Koutouzow Tolstoy.
Tolstoy's Letters selected, ed. and tr. R. F. Christian.
Tolstoy, Leo *War and Peace* tr. Louise and Aylmer Maude.
Tolstoy, Count Lev. N. *What Is Art?* tr. Leo Wiener.
Tolstoy, Count Lev. N. *What Shall We Do Then?* tr. Leo Wiener.
Tolstoy's Writings on Civil Disobedience and Non-Violence Bergman Publishers.
Troyat, Henri *Tolstoy* tr. Nancy Amphoux.

14. Mahatma Gandhi's Nonviolent Revolution
Ashe, Geoffrey *Gandhi.*
Bondurant, Joan V. *Conquest of Violence:* The Gandhian Philosophy of Conflict.
Easwaran, Eknath *Gandhi the Man.*
Erikson, Erik H. *Gandhi's Truth:* On the Origins of Militant Nonviolence.

Fischer, Louis *Gandhi:* His Life and Message for the World.

Fischer, Louis *The Life of Mahatma Gandhi.*

Gandhi, Mahatma *All Men Are Brothers:* Autobiographical Reflections.

Gandhi, Mohandas K. *An Autobiography:* The Story of My Experiments With Truth.

Gandhi, Mahatma *Hind Swaraj or Indian Home Rule.*

Gandhi, M. K. *Nonviolent Resistance (Satyagraha).*

Gandhi, M. K. *For Pacifists.*

Iyer, Raghavan *The Moral and Political Thought of Mahatma Gandhi.*

Lewis, Martin Deming (ed.) *Gandhi: Maker of Modern India:*

Mehta, Ved *Mahatma Gandhi and His Apostles.*

Ramachandran, G. and Mahadevan, T. K. (ed.) *Gandhi: His Relevance for Our Times.*

Ray, Sibnarayan (ed.) *Gandhi, India and the World:* An International Symposium.

Rolland, Romain *Mahatma Gandhi:* The Man Who Became One with the Universal Being, tr. Catherine D. Groth.

Sheean, Vincent *Lead, Kindly Light:* Gandhi & the Way to Peace.

Shirer, William L. *Gandhi: A Memoir.*

Wellock, Wilfred *India's Social Revolution led by Mahatma Gandhi and now Vinoba Bhave.*

15. Woodrow Wilson and the League of Nations

Aurobindo *War and Self-Determination.*

Bailey, Thomas A. *Woodrow Wilson and the Lost Peace.*

Bailey, Thomas A. *Woodrow Wilson and the Great Betrayal.*

Baker, Ray Stannard *Woodrow Wilson and World Settlement* 3 Volumes.

Bendiner, Elmer *A Time For Angels:* The Tragicomic History of the League of Nations.

Blum, John Morton *Woodrow Wilson and the Politics of Morality.*

Clemenceau, Georges *Grandeur and Misery of Victory.*

Cranston, Alan *The Killing of the Peace.*

Dos Passos, John *Mr. Wilson's War.*

Eaton, W. D. and Harry C. Read *Woodrow Wilson: His Life and Work.*

Foley, Hamilton *Woodrow Wilson's Case for the League of Nations.*

Freud, Sigmund and William C. Bullitt *Thomas Woodrow Wilson:* A Psychological Study.

Garraty, John A. *Woodrow Wilson.*

George, Alexander L. and Juliette L. George *Woodrow Wilson and Colonel House:* A Personality Study.

Harley, J. Eugene *Woodrow Wilson Still Lives — His World Ideals Triumphant.*

Hoover, Herbert *The Ordeal of Woodrow Wilson.*

Ions, Edmund *Woodrow Wilson:* The Politics of Peace and War.

Levin, N. Gordon *Woodrow Wilson and World Politics.*

Link, Arthur S. *Woodrow Wilson:* A Brief Biography.

Mayer, Arno J. *Politics and Diplomacy of Peacemaking:* Containment and Counterrevolution at Versailles 1918-1919.

Mee, Charles L., Jr. *The End of Order:* Versailles 1919.

Seymour, Charles (ed.) *The Intimate Papers of Colonel House* 4 Volumes.

Smith, Gene *When the Cheering Stopped:* the last years of Woodrow Wilson.

Tumulty, Joseph P. *Woodrow Wilson As I Know Him.*

Waller, Bolton C. *Paths to World-Peace.*

Walters, F. P. *A History of the League of Nations* 2 Volumes

White, William Allen *Woodrow Wilson.*

Wilson, Edith Bolling *My Memoir.*

Wilson: Great Lives Observed, ed. John Braeman.

Wilson, Woodrow *The State:* Elements of Historical and Practical Politics.

Woodrow Wilson's Own Story ed. Donald Day.

16. Franklin Roosevelt and the United Nations

Bailey, Sydney D. *The United Nations:* A Short Political Guide.

Bishop, Jim *FDR's Last Year.*

Boyd, Andrew *Fifteen Men on a Powder Keg:* A History of the U. N. Security Council.

Building Peace: Reports of the Commission to Study the Organization of Peace 1939-1972, 2 Vols.

Burns, James MacGregor *Roosevelt: The Lion and the Fox 1882-1940.*

Burns, James MacGregor *Roosevelt: The Soldier of Freedom 1940-1945.*

Campbell, Thomas M. *Madquerade Peace:* America's UN Policy, 1944-1945.

Claude, Inis L., Jr. *The Changing United Nations.*

Claude, Inis L., Jr. *Swords into Plowshares:* The Problems and Progress of International Organization.

Churchill, Winston S. *Closing the Ring:* The Second World War, Vol. 5.

Churchill, Winston S. *The Grand Alliance:* The Second World War, Vol. 3

Churchill, Winston S. *Triumph and Tragedy:* The Second World War, Vol. 6.

Coyle, David Cushman *The United Nations and How It Works.*

Dallek, Robert *Franklin D. Roosevelt and American Foreign Policy, 1932-1945.*

de Arechaga, Eduardo Jiminez *Voting and the Handling of Disputes in the Security Council.*

de Sa, Hernane Tavares *The Play Within the Play:* The Inside Story of the UN.

Eichelberger, Clark M. *Organizing for Peace:* A Personal History of the Founding of the United Nations.

Everyman's United Nations: A Complete Handbook of trhe Activities and Evolution of the United Nations During its First Twenty Years.

Forsythe, David P. *United Nations Peacemaking:* The Conciliation Commission for Palestine.

Goodrich, Leland M. and Anne P. Simons *The United Nations and the Maintenance of International Peace and Security.*

Gunther, John *Roosevelt in Retrospect.*

Hammerskjold, Dag *Markings* tr. Leif Sjoberg and W. H. Auden.

Lash, Joseph P. *Eleanor and Franklin.*

Malik, Charles *Man in the Struggle for Peace.*

Neilson, Winthrop and Frances *The United Nations: The World's Last Chance for Peace.*

Nicholas, H. G. *The United Nations as a Political Institution.*

Peace on Earth Intro. by Robert Sherwood.

Perkins, Frances *The Roosevelt I Knew.*

Roosevelt, Eleanor *This I Remember.*

Roosevelt, Eleanor and William De Witt *UN: Today and Tomorrow.*

Roosevelt, Elliott *As He Saw It.*

Roosevelt, Franklin D. *Looking Forward.*

Nothing to Fear: The Selected Addresses of Franklin Delano Roosevelt 1932-1945.

Franklin D. Roosevelt's Own Story ed. Donald Day.

Ross, Alf *The United Nations: Peace and Progress.*

Sherwood, Robert E. *Roosevelt and Hopkins:* An Intimate History.

Soderberg, Sten *Hammerskjold.*

Stone, Julius *Conflict Through Consensus:* United Nations Approaches to Aggression.

Truman, Harry S. *Memoirs: Year of Decisions.*

Truman, Harry S. *Memoirs: Years of Trial and Hope 1946-1952.*

Tully, Grace *F. D. R. My Boss.*

The United Nations and Human Rights: Eighteenth Report of the Commission to Study the Organization of Peace.

Wainhouse, David W. *International Peacekeeping at the Crossroads.*

Wainhouse, David W. *International Peace Observation.*

Welles, Sumner *The Time for Decision.*

17. Einstein and Schweitzer on Peace in the Atomic Age

Anderson, Erica *Albert Schweitzer's Gift of Friendship.*

Barnett, Lincoln *The Universe and Dr. Einstein.*

Beckhard, Arthur *Albert Einstein.*

Calder, Nigel *Einstein's Universe.*

Clark, Ronald W. *Einstein: The Life and Times.*

Cousins, Norman *Dr. Schweitzer of Lambaréné.*

Cuny, Hilaire *Albert Einstein: The Man and His Theories* tr. Mervyn Savill.

de Broglie, Louis et al *Einstein* tr. Peebles Press International

Albert Einstein: The Human Side ed. Helen Dukas and Banesh Hoffman.

Einstein on Peace ed. Otto Nathan and Heinz Norden.

Einstein, Albert *Ideas and Opinions* tr. Sonja Bargmann.

Einstein, Albert *Out of My Later Years.*

Einstein, Albert *Relativity: The Special and the General Theory* tr. Robert W. Lawson.

Einstein, Albert *The World As I See It* tr. Alan Harris.

Feschotte, Jacques *Albert Schweitzer: An Introduction* tr. John Russell.

Kraus, Oskar *Albert Schweitzer: His Work and His Philosophy* tr. E. G. McCalman.

Marshall, George and David Poling *Schweitzer: A Biography.*

Payne, Robert *The Three Worlds of Albert Schweitzer.*

Picht, Werner *Albert Schweitzer: The Man and His Work* tr. Edward Fitzgerald.

Roback, A. A. (ed.) *The Albert Schweitzer Jubilee Book.*

Albert Schweitzer: An Anthology ed. Charles R. Joy.

Schweitzer, Albert *Indian Thought and Its Development* tr. Mrs. C. E. B. Russell.

Schweitzer, Albert *Out of My Life and Thought: An Autobiography* tr. C. T. Campion.

Schweitzer, Albert *Peace or Atomic War?*

Schweitzer, Albert *The Philosophy of Civilization* tr. C. T. Campion.

Schweitzer, Albert *Reverence for Life* tr. Reginald H. Fuller.

The Wisdom of Albert Schweitzer.

Seaver, George *Albert Schweitzer: The Man and His Mind.*

18. The Pacifism of Bertrand Russell and A. J. Muste

Brock, Peter *Twentieth-Century Pacifism.*

Chatfield, Charles (ed.) *Peace Movements in America.*

Clark, Ronald W. *The Life of Bertrand Russell.*

Cooney, Robert and Helen Michalowski *The Power of the People: Active Nonviolence in the United States.*

Hentoff, Nat *Peace Agitator: The Story of A. J. Muste.*

The Essays of A. J. Muste ed. by Nat Hentoff.

Muste, A. J. *Nonviolence in an Aggressive World.*

Russell, Bertrand *The ABC of Relativity.*

Russell, Bertrand *The Art of Philosophizing and Other Essays.*

The Autobiography of Bertrand' Russell: The Early Years: 1872-World War I.

The Autobiography of Bertrand Russell: The Middle Years: 1914-1944.

The Autobiography of Bertrand Russell: The Final Years: 1944-1969.

The Basic Writings of Bertrand Russell.

Russell, Bertrand *Common Sense and Nuclear Warfare.*

Russell, Bertrand *The Conquest of Happiness.*

Russell, Bertrand *Education and the Good Life.*

Russell, Bertrand *Essays in Analysis* ed. by Douglas Lackey.

Russell, Bertrand *Fact and Fiction.*

Russell, Bertrand *Has Man a Future?*

Russell, Bertrand *A History of Western Philosophy.*

Russell, Bertrand *Human Society in Ethics and Politics.*

Russell, Bertrand *The Impact of Science on Society.*

Russell, Bertrand *An Inquiry into Meaning and Truth.*

Russell, Bertrand *Justice in War Time.*

Russell, Bertrand *Marriage and Morals.*

Russell, Bertrand *New Hopes for a Changing World.*

Russell, Bertrand *Nightmares of Eminent Persons and Other Stories.*

Russell, Bertrand *Political Ideals.*

Russell, Bertrand *Power.*

Russell, Bertrand *The Problems of Philosophy.*

Russell, Bertrand and Dora Russell *The Prospects of Industrial Civilization.*

Russell, Bertrand *Religion and Science.*
Russell, Bertrand *Roads to Freedom.*
Russell, Bertrand *Sceptical Essays.*
Russell, Bertrand *The Scientific Outlook.*
Bertrand Russell Speaks His Mind.
Russell, Bertrand *Unarmed Victory.*
Russell, Bertrand *Unpopular Essays.*
Russell, Bertrand *War Crimes in Vietnam.*
Russell, Bertrand *Which Way to Peace?*
Russell, Bertrand *Why I Am Not a Christian.*
Russell, Bertrand *Why Men Fight.*
Russell, Bertrand *The Will to Doubt.*
Russell, Bertrand *Wisdom of the West.*
Whitehead, Alfred North and Bertrand Russell *Principia Mathematica.*

19. Martin Luther King and the Civil Rights Movement

Garrow, David J. *The FBI and Martin Luther King, Jr.*
Lewis, David L. *King: A Critical Biography.*
King, Coretta Scott *My Life with Martin Luther King, Jr.*
King, Martin Luther Jr. *Stride Toward Freedom.*
King, Martin Luther Jr. *Where Do We Go from Here: Chaos or Community?*
King, Martin Luther Jr. *Why We Can't Wait.*
Peck, Ira *The Life and Words of Martin Luther King, Jr.*
Smith, George H. *Martin Luther King Jr.*

20. Lessons of Vietnam

Ashmore, Harry S. and William C. Baggs *Mission to Hanoi.*
Brown, Sam and Len Ackland (Ed.) *Why Are We Still in Vietnam?*
Chomsky, Noam *At War with Asia.*
Chomsky, Noam *For Reasons of State.*
Chomsky, Noam and Edward S. Herman *The Political Economy of Human Rights* (2 Volumes) I: *The Washington Connection and Third World Fascism* and II: *After the Cataclysm: Postwar Indochina and the Reconstruction of Imperial Ideology.*
Cooper, Chester *The Lost Crusade.*
Draper, Theodore *Abuse of Power.*

Ellsberg, Daniel *Papers on the War.*

Falk, Richard A. (Ed.) *The Vietnam War and International Law.*

Fitzgerald, Frances *Fire in the Lake.*

Gettleman, Marvin E. (Ed.) *Vietnam: History, Documents, and Opinions on a Major World Crisis.*

Grant, Jonathan S., Laurence A. G. Moss, and Jonathan Unger *Cambodia: The Widening War in Indochina.*

Halberstam, David *The Best and the Brightest.*

Halstead, Fred *Out Now: A Participant's Account of the American Movement Against the Vietnam War.*

Hanh, Thich Nhat *Vietnam: Lotus in a Sea of Fire.*

Kahin, George McTurnan and John W. Lewis *The United States in Vietnam.*

Knoll, Erwin and Judith Nies McFadden (Ed.) *War Crimes and the American Conscience.*

Kraslow, David and Stuart H. Loory *The Secret Search for Peace in Vietnam.*

Ky, Nguyen Cao *How We Lost the Vietnam War.*

Lacouture, Jean *Vietnam: Between Two Truces* tr. Konrad Kellen and Joel Carmichael.

Lynd, Staughton and Thomas Hayden *The Other Side.*

Peace in Vietnam: A Report Prepared for the American Friends Service Committee.

Pfeffer, Richard M. (Ed.) *No More Vietnams?*

Porter, Gareth (Ed.) *Vietnam: A History in Documents.*

Raskin, Marcus G. and Bernard B. Fall *The Viet-Nam Reader.*

Reischauer, Edwin O. *Beyond Vietnam.*

Russell, Bertrand *War Crimes in Vietnam.*

Salisbury, Harrison E. *Behind the Lines — Hanoi.*

Santoli, Al *Everything We Had.*

Schlesinger, Arthur M. Jr. *The Bitter Heritage.*

Schurmann, Franz, Peter Dale Scott, and Reginald Zelnik *The Politics of Escalation in Vietnam.*

Shawcross, William *Side-show: Kissinger, Nixon and the Destruction of Cambodia.*

Sheehan, Neil *The Pentagon Papers.*

Smith, Ralph *Viet-Nam and the West.*

Tanham, George K. *War Without Guns.*

Taylor, Telford *Nuremberg and Vietnam: An American Tragedy.*

The Vietnam Hearings.

White, Ralph K. *Nobody Wanted War.*

Woodstone, Norma Sue *Up Against the War.*

Zagoria, Donald S. *Vietnam Triangle: Moscow, Peking, Hanoi.*

Zinn, Howard *Vietnam: The Logic of Withdrawal.*

21. The Clark-Sohn Proposal for World Law and Disarmament

Barnet, Richard J. *Who Wants Disarmament.*

Brenna, Donald G. (ed.) *Arms Control, Disarmament, and National Security.*

Brierly, J. L. *The Law of Nations* ed. by Humphrey Waldock.

Clark, Grenville *A Plan for Peace.*

Clark, Grenville and Louis Sohn *Introduction to World Peace Through World Law* revised by Louis Sohn, 1973.

Clark, Grenville and Louis B. Sohn *World Peace Through World Law* Second Edition (Revised).

Claude, Inis L. Jr. *Swords Into Plowshares: The Problems and Progress of International Organization.*

Collins, Edward Jr. *International Law in a Changing World.*

Cousins, Norman *In Place of Folly.*

Cousins, Norman *Modern Man Is Obsolete.*

Etzioni, Amitai *The Hard Way to Peace.*

Falk, Richard A. and Saul H. Mendlovitz (ed.). *The Strategy of World Order:* Volume 1 *Toward a Theory of War Prevention,* Volume 2 *International Law,* Volume 3 *The United Nations,* Volume 4 *Disarmament and Economic Development.*

Falk, Richard A. *A Study of Future Worlds.*

Falk, Richard, Samuel S. Kim, and Saul H. Mendlovitz (ed.) *Toward a Just World Order.*

Fenwick, Charles G. *International Law.*

Gardner, Richard N. (ed.) *Blueprint for Peace.*

Johansen, Robert C. *The National Interest and the Human Interest.*

Johnson, Andrew N. *Enforceable World Peace.*

Lissitzyn, Oliver J. *The International Court of Justice.*

Mendlovitz, Saul H. (ed.) *Legal and Political Problems of World Order.*

Mendlovitz, Saul H. (ed). *On the Creation of a Just World Order.*

Millis, Walter and James Real *The Abolition of War.*

Mische, Gerald and Patricia *Toward a Human World Order.*

Nuclear Weapons: Report of the Secretary-General of the United Nations.

Ramundo, Bernard A. *Peaceful Coexistence: International Law in the Building of Communism.*

Reves, Emery *The Anatomy of Peace.*

Wainhouse, David W. *International Peacekeeping at the Crossroads.*

Wainhouse, David W. *Arms Control Agreements: Designs for Verification and Organization.*

Wilson, Bernard John *Universal Evolution and the Road to Peace.*

Wright, Quincy, William M. Evan and Morton Deutsch (ed.) *Preventing World War III: Some Proposals.*

Ziegler, David W. *War, Peace, and International Politics.*

22. Women and Peace

Addams, Jane *A Centennial Reader.*

Addams, Jane *Forty Years at Hull-house.*

Addams, Jane *Newer Ideals of Peace.*

Addams, Jane *The Overthrow of the War System.*

Addams, Jane *Patriotism and Pacifists in War Time.*

Addams, Jane *Peace and Bread in Time of War.*

Artus, Marjorie and Louis C. Line *The New Age: The New Woman.*

Boulding, Elise *The Underside of History.*

Bussey, Gertrude and Margaret Tims *Pioneers for Peace: Women's International League for Peace and Freedom 1915-1965.*

Catt, Carrie Chapman and Nettie Rogers Shuler *Women Suffrage and Politics.*

Cooney, Robert and Helen Michalowski *The Power of the People.*

Day, Dorothy *Loaves and Fishes.*
Day, Dorothy *The Long Loneliness.*
Day, Dorothy *On Pilgrimage: The Sixties.*
Degen, Marie Louise *The History of the Woman's Peace Party.*
Deming, Barbara *On Anger/New Men New Women.*
Deming, Barbara *Revolution & Equilibrium.*
Dworkin, Andrea *Our Blood.*
Eastman, Crystal *On Women and Revolution.*
Lerner, Gerda *The Grimke Sisters from South Carolina.*
Liberation Now! Writings from the Women's Liberation Movement.
McAllister, Pam (ed.) *Reweaving the Web of Life: Feminism and Nonviolence.*
Miller, William D. *Dorothy Day.*
Montagu, Ashley *The Natural Superiority of Women.*
O'Neill, William L. *Everyone Was Brave: A History of Feminism in America.*
Sivard, Ruth *World Military and Social Expenditures 1982.*
Starhawk *Dreaming the Dark: Magic, Sex & Politics.*
Women of Europe in Action for Peace called by Women's International League for Peace and Freedom.
World Congress of Women — Equality, National Independence, Peace.

23. The Anti-Nuclear Movement
Adams, Ruth and Susan Cullen (ed.) *The Final Epidemic: Physicians and Scientists on Nuclear War.*
Aldridge, Robert C. *First Strike!*
Barash, David P. and Judith Eve Lipton *Stop Nuclear War!*
Building United Judgment: A Handbook for Consensus Decision Making.
Calder, Nigel *Nuclear Nightmares.*
Caldicott, Helen *Nuclear Madness.*
Common Security: A Blueprint for Survival by the Independent Commission on Disarmament and Security Issues.
Creating Peace: A Positive Handbook.
Curtis, Richard and Elizabeth Hogan *Nuclear Lessons.*
Day, Samuel H. Jr. "The New Resistance" *The Progressive* April 1983.
Diablo Canyon Blockade/Encampment Handbook.

Dietrich, Jeff *Reluctant Resister.*

Direct Action Mid-July 1983.

Freeze It? a citizen's guide to reversing the nuclear arms race.

Ground Zero July/August 1983.

Ground Zero *Nuclear War: What's in it For You?*

Ground Zero *What About the Russians and Nuclear War?*

Gyorgy, Anna and friends *No Nukes.*

Harvest of Justice July 1983.

International Day of Nuclear Disarmament.

Kaplan, David E. (ed.) *Nuclear California.*

Kaplan, Fred *The Wizards of Armageddon.*

Kennan, George F. *The Nuclear Delusion.*

Kennedy, Edward M. and Mark O. Hatfield *Freeze!*

Keyes, Ken Jr. *The Hundredth Monkey.*

Lefever, Ernest W. and E. Stephen Hunt (ed.) *The Apocalyptic Premise.*

Lifton, Robert Jay and Richard Falk *Indefensible Weapons.*

Lovins, Amory B. and L. Hunter Lovins *Energy/War: Breaking the Nuclear Link.*

Martin, Laurence (ed.) *Strategic Thought in the Nuclear Age.*

Nuclear Times August/September 1983.

Nuclear Weapons: Report of the Secretary-General.

Questions & Answers on the Soviet Threat and National Security.

Reader, Mark (ed.) *Atom's Eve: Ending the Nuclear Age.*

Scheer, Robert *With Enough Shovels: Reagan, Bush & Nuclear War.*

Schell, Jonathan *The Fate of the Earth.*

Stanley, C. Maxwell *Multilateral Disarmament: Conspiracy for Common Sense.*

Synthesis August 1983.

Thompson, E. P. *Beyond the Cold War.*

Thompson, E. P. and Dan Smith (ed.) *Protest and Survive.*

The Vandenberg Action: A Handbook for Nonviolent Direct Action.

Wallis, Jim (ed.) *Waging Peace.*

You Can Prevent Nuclear War (Common Cause).

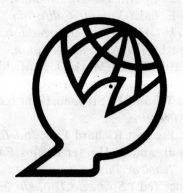

WORLD PEACE MOVEMENT

Evolving Principles, Purposes, and Methods

The World Peace Movement is a response to the longing of millions of people for peace on earth. The death and destruction caused by wars, the threat of mass annihilation by nuclear war, and the misappropriation of vast amounts of human, technical, and financial resources for an insatiable arms race have aroused cries of protest.

The World Peace Movement is a positive process leading to enduring solutions to the problems of war, militarism, and a lawless world. We consider the need for world peace to be the first priority of human civilization and essential to the continued development of the human race.

The World Peace Movement is endeavoring to facilitate the action of all people in every country who are working for world peace.

Principles

1. The earth is one world, and its human beings must learn to live in peace with each other or perish.
2. The human race is one and interdependent; the good of each depends on the good of all and our love for each other.
3. The way of love and peace is non-violent and does not hurt anyone.
4. The uniting power of love, peace, and friendship is stronger than the divisive strife of hatred, war, and enmity.
5. The conversion of a hostile and militaristic world into a peaceful global society is primarily an educational process of changing consciousness from fear, suspicion, and mistrust to love, confidence, and trust in the human capacity to solve problems, cooperate, and establish justice.
6. Every human being has the equal right to life, liberty, security, and justice.
7. Respect for individual freedom and dignity requires the protection of all human rights by means of a universal system of justice.

279

8. Justice in human affairs evolves through democratic means and due process of law.

9. The use of force is justified only when a legal authority, designated by consent of the people, is required to restrain and bring to justice a violator of the law.

10. A law enforcement official has legal authority only within the territory of the people who designate that official. No nation has the sovereign right to use any force outside its national borders.

11. War, the use of force outside one's territory, the threat to use such force, and the sale or transfer of military weapons outside one's territory should be prohibited by international law.

12. International wars and internal oppression of human rights are allowed to occur because there is no enforceable world law.

13. Enforceable world law and justice may be established by instituting a democratically elected federal world government to protect human rights and solve international disputes through a compulsory system of jurisprudence.

14. In a federal world government each nation would maintain sovereignty over its own internal affairs, except that the federal world government would have legal authority to protect human rights and settle international disputes.

15. Education, communication, democratic process, and nonviolent protest of wrongs are the purest and most effective means of social reform. Peace and justice are attained only by peaceful and just means.

16. Biological, chemical, and nuclear weapons are so horrendously deadly to people and damaging to the environment for such long periods of time that only deluded minds seriously contemplate their use.

17. Belief in deterrence of war by massive armaments and nuclear weapons is based on fear, suspicion, mistrust, and insecurity; this weapons policy perpetrates more fear, suspicion, mistrust, and insecurity in the world.

18. Those people who have moral courage and faith in the justice of their economic and political philosophies and in the nonviolent social change of democratic processes will support enforceable world law instead of massive national armaments.

19. Huge expenditures on massive armaments of destruction are a colossal waste of human and material resources, causing poverty, inflation, and a lowering of the quality of life. Such resources could otherwise be used for improvement of the environment, food production and distribution, education, health, and other beneficial purposes.

Purposes

1. To awaken the inner peace that dwells in the hearts of all beings.

2. To create the consciousness of world peace and to foster friendship and harmony among all people.

3. To promote and protect the human rights of all people, regardless of race, color, sex, language, religion, political or other opinion, national or social origin, property, birth or other status, as delineated in the Universal Declaration of Human Rights of the United Nations.

4. To assure international justice and universal human rights by developing ways to preserve them, such as a federal world government, democratically elected by all the people of the earth, with a world court of justice having compulsory jurisdiction to decide all cases of international disputes and violations of world law and human rights, and with a world peacekeeping force of individuals from all countries who would be dedicated to the whole of humanity and who would enforce world law and the decisions of the world court of justice by the most peaceful means possible.

5. To achieve disarmament and the total elimination of all biological, chemical, and nuclear weapons in the entire world.

6. To purify and maintain a clean and ecologically balanced environment for our health and prosperity and for future generations.

7. To alleviate poverty and hunger, and to improve the health, education, and living conditions of all people on earth.

8. To encourage all schools from the primary grades to the university to offer peace education from a global perspective.

Methods

1. To live peacefully and lovingly as examples to all.
2. To educate ourselves and others by every means to increase awareness of the oneness of life, the interdependence of all beings, the ecological unity of the environment, the way of love and nonviolence, and the urgent need for transnational attitudes, programs, and institutions for the sake of mutual survival.
3. To communicate by every means the truth and the facts which reveal and nourish world peace.
4. To pray and meditate and expand the consciousness of peace.
5. To respect and nurture human rights with tolerance and understanding.
6. To refrain from contributing to the preparations and activities of war and from hostile and aggressive attitudes.
7. To protest nonviolently against oppression, militarism, nuclear weapons, pollution, and violations of human rights.
8. To work for the total elimination of biological, chemical, and nuclear weapons in every country.
9. To promote and practice world citizenship, and to work to organize a world constitutional convention to plan the democratic institution of a federal world government.
10. To use all human wisdom, sciences, and technologies in developing and purifying the environment, eradicating hunger and sickness in all countries, and making global education available to all people.
11. To communicate closely with all peace organizations and dedicated peace workers to facilitate the forming of a united worldwide network to bring about the establishment of world peace.

World Peace Movement
P.O. Box 2
Ojai, CA 93023
USA

Please contact the peace organization in your area for information about local activities.

"Think globally, and act locally."

282

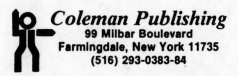

Coleman Publishing
99 Milbar Boulevard
Farmingdale, New York 11735
(516) 293-0383-84